This book is dedicated to all the people out there who are struggling with infertility, I hope I can make you laugh today!

HILARIOUSLY INFERTILE

ONE WOMAN'S INAPPROPRIATE QUEST TO HELP WOMEN LAUGH THROUGH INFERTILITY

KAREN JEFFRIES

Hilariously Infertile

Print ISBN: 978-1-54393-766-4
eBook ISBN: 978-1-54393-767-1

TABLE OF CONTENTS

CHAPTER 1

My Name is Karen and I am Infertile

Hello Ladies! (Oh and hello to the few "supportive" men who were bullied into reading this book). I am infertile and no one likes to talk about it. If you are infertile, you are not alone. Let me start at the beginning, I was born on…HA! Just kidding, that book would **suck**. No, let's start at the other beginning. Soon after we were engaged, my husband and I moved in together in the fall of 2009. My husband, John, proposed after we jumped out of a plane together. *Yeah, we are those cool people.* We were married in August of 2010. I had no plans of starting a family anytime soon. I told people, including myself, that I wanted to wait until I was thirty-five to start "trying." Well, I am turning thirty-four in a week and I have a dog, two kids and a house in the suburbs, so that plan sure as heck went to hell in a handbasket and **fast**.

We went to pick up our dog in June of 2010. That was when the motherhood juices really started flowing. We were towards the end of our engagement; the wedding was right around the corner. Brady, our Australian Labradoodle love of our lives, was the perfect thing for us. I tell people that Brady is my first-born child. I truly believe that he thinks I pushed him out of my vagina, and to be honest, if you saw the way we spoon each other at nighttime, you would think so too.

I trained Brady over the summer. I would play with him on the floor of our living room because he was too little to jump onto the couch. Then, he would fall asleep on my lap for two hours and I would be stuck there, on the living room floor, under my sleeping puppy. When he awoke, I would carry him on my hip, like a child, to my elevator and take him for a walk. If I did not carry him, he would pee a little in the elevator. When I did carry him, he would pee a little on my shirt and make it look like I was a lactating mother, but I didn't mind. Brady was my child.

I had a little bag of training treats attached to my pants and a clicker to house train him. Once, in the elevator, someone asked me if I was the dog trainer.

"Oh no," I said, "I'm just neurotic about training him."

When he went for his first haircut, which turned out to be a disaster, I cried for two days straight. John called the dog salon and made them refund us the money because he could not listen to me sob about Brady's hair any longer. Brady was my child.

We were a very happily married couple. I liked being married and not having kids. Brady was plenty for me. I liked living in NYC and getting drunk on the weekends. I really liked sleeping in late and ordering bagels delivered. Then, when the sun got to the right spot in the sky, I really liked ordering wine delivered and starting the whole cycle over again. It was perfect. I did not need kids. However hearing John tell Brady, "Go get Mommy," totally made those Mommy emotions twinge.

In June of 2011, my best friend told me she was pregnant. A few weeks later, my sister told me that she was pregnant. Correction, I told my sister that I thought she was pregnant – we will get to that. Regardless, that is when I started getting the "pregnancy bug."

What is it? Why is it that when women get pregnant and have babies it makes other women want to get pregnant and have babies? Why? It's not as if they have a Louis Vuitton purse and I, too, would like one. Well, let's be real, I'm a school teacher. So in my case, it would be more as if they have a Michael Kors purse and I, too, want a Michael Kors purse. (To the five men who were bullied into reading this book please pause and ask your bully what that means…you back? Great!)

My best friend, who we are going to call Shamecha because that name is **awesome**, and I were on our way to a bridal shower for another friend. She wanted me to come to her apartment and drive to the bridal shower together. She was insistent on this. I could not understand why. It was not making sense. We kept texting back and forth about it and finally I gave in. I pulled into the parking lot of her apartment. We moved her car so that I could park mine in her spot. I was putting my bridal shower present in the back of her car when I saw a CVS Pharmacy bag full of pregnancy tests and tampons.

"Uhhh, are you pregnant?" I asked, positive that the answer would be no.

"Yeah, I am," she said. "And you're messing this all up, we were supposed to drive together and I was supposed to tell you in the car, but now you saw the bag and, yeah, I'm pregnant!"

She had the biggest smile on her face. "OH MY GOD!!!!" I squealed, as I gave her a huge hug. We talked about her pregnancy and the way she felt the whole way to the bridal shower. Once we got to the shower, we were surrounded by things that she could not eat or drink: coffee, mimosas, soft cheese, and the list went on. After the shower, we drove to Barnes and Noble and I bought her a number of pregnancy books to read because neither one of us knew what to do when you are pregnant.

A few weeks later, my sister called me just to talk. My sister, who was married that April, went off the pill at the end of May. It was June. She started telling me about all of these random symptoms she was having and how she was sure that she was going to get her period any day now, but how it had not come yet.

"What type of symptoms?" I asked her suspiciously.

"Well, like, my boobs hurt, a lot. I'm tired. I don't know. I just want these symptoms to go away and my period to come already," she said.

My sister, who is perfectly balanced equal parts smart/not smart, did not know what was happening.

"Kate, how long have you had these symptoms?" I asked, as if I was asking a student about missing homework.

"Umm, well, for about two weeks now, I think," she said in her not smart talk.

"Kate, your period is not going to come you dumb fuck, you're pregnant!" I said.

"No, I really don't think so," she tried to convince me.

After significant back and forth, she agreed to go buy some pregnancy tests. She called me back two hours later.

"Umm… so, I think I'm pregnant," she said.

"You think? What does that mean, you think?" I questioned aggressively.

"Well, I took two pregnancy tests and they both came back positive, so I think that means I'm pregnant," the not smart part of her continued.

"You **think** that means you're pregnant? Kate this is not a 'you **think**' situation. You are freaking pregnant!"

"Yeah, I am," she conceded.

My sister's pregnancy went off without a hitch – kind of – we will get to that. My best friend's pregnancy, however, was not on the same track.

Shamecha suffered a miscarriage eight weeks into her pregnancy. She was devastated and so was I. I was so excited for her to be pregnant. I had been checking in on her every day to see how she felt.

It was June, Field Day. All teachers hate Field Day, except for the PE teachers who run and organize it. Prior to the invention of black workout pants, Field Day was actual torture. Let's take all these women who do not know what to wear, and put them onto a field so they can awkwardly sweat through their shirts and pants. Nothing says "school spirit" like bra and crotch sweat. Shamecha did not technically have to partake in Field Day. I walked into her room that morning.

"How are you feeling today?" I asked with a smile.

"Weird," she said.

"But like normal weird right?" I asked.

"No, not normal weird. I feel very crampy," she said as she looked up at the ceiling and fluffed her hair away from her face with both hands.

"Well, cramping is normal this early on, isn't it?" I asked, not even thinking about the alternative.

"I think so, but this feels different. I'm taking a half-day and going home," she said.

"I'm sure it's nothing, but good. You should. Go rest. I'll call you after work." I smiled and left her room, thinking nothing of it.

That afternoon my grade level was hosting a First Grade Orientation meeting for parents of current kindergarten students who would be in first grade in September. It was a meeting to explain the expectations of first grade to them, which they did not believe, understand, nor respect.

After the meeting, I got in my car to drive home. I saw a missed call from Shamecha, and, instead of listening to the voicemail, I just called her right away. She did not pick up. I left a message complaining about Field Day and the orientation meeting. Then, I checked the message that she left me as I was getting on I-95 south.

"Hey, it's me," she started, "so I had a miscarriage. I'm okay. I'm going home. I just wanted you to know."

I gasped aloud. My heart sank to my stomach. I started breathing heavy; tears were welling up in my eyes, making driving nearly impossible. I called her back immediately. I left yet another voicemail apologizing profusely for not listening to her message first, and for not being able to pick up the phone in the first place because of my stupid first grade meeting. I drove the whole way home to the city with foggy, cloudy, tear-covered eyes. When I got home, I cried into my labradoodle pillow, and then worse when we actually spoke on the phone that night.

Her miscarriage hit me hard. How could my best friend, and a perfectly healthy girl, suffer a miscarriage? If it could happen to her, could it happen to anyone? This was all new to me, but it scared the shit out of me. I wanted to start "trying" to get pregnant with my husband, and why not pull the goalie? (Pull the goalie is a colloquial term meaning to go off the pill that had been preventing me from getting pregnant for about ten years.) I was in no rush to get pregnant.

The whole subject of "trying" to get pregnant is such a hoax. Any woman who is "trying" to get pregnant, or doing the whole, "we are just not stopping it from happening anymore," is full of shit. The second a woman starts, "trying," to get pregnant she officially wants to **be** pregnant. The minute she takes her first pregnancy test and it is negative, but she was hoping it would be positive, her mind is made up. She wants to be pregnant and she wants it – **yesterday**.

CHAPTER 2

"Trying"

I WENT ON THE PILL WHEN I WAS 19 YEARS OLD, A FRESHMAN IN college. I had been sexually active before that, but I always used condoms. Now, I was dating some guy who wanted me on the pill. He was clever about it too. We had sex and then he told me that we could not have any more sex if I did not go on the pill. I was horny. So when I was home from school one vacation, I lied to my parents, went to Planned Parenthood, and started on birth control. I paid for the appointment and the pills by myself so my parents wouldn't know. The sex was mediocre, for the record.

Fast forward two years later and I was in a somewhat serious relationship – as serious as a relationship can be when you are twenty years old. I was home from college and my mother and I were in the car. She started talking about sex and the pill. MORTIFYING!!! She said things like, "I'm a cool Mom," and, "I think it's time we put you on the pill."

What is that taste in my mouth? Oh, it is vomit; I just vomited in my mouth a little and swallowed it back down. All I heard was *blah, blah, blah, I will pay for your birth control from now on.*

Yes please! Sign me up!

She never knew that I was on the pill prior to that. Well, until now, sorry Mom.

So, as I said, I had been on the pill for about a decade. After a lot of conversation, and my husband pushing back, he finally gave in. We decided that we were going to stop the pill and just "see what happens" (again total bullshit because the minute that we decided to start "trying" to get pregnant I already wanted to be pregnant). It was July 2011. I was hoping I would get pregnant quickly because I'm a school teacher and I wanted to **plan** it so I could have a spring baby, take my maternity leave, and go back to work in September without disruption.

My first real pearl of wisdom for girls trying to get pregnant is: forget the calendar. Do not try to **plan** what month you will give birth. It just will not happen. It is a pointless activity and it will only lead you to stress out when you realize that you missed your, "optimal birth month window," which, by the way, there is no "optimal birth month window." It will happen when it happens and it will totally rock the shit out of your world for both good and for bad, regardless of which month it happens.

We were officially "trying." We were having unprotected sex all the time. Weeks and months went by and I was not getting my period. So I was pregnant, right? I was having a lot of unprotected sex, putting pillows under my ass after it. Sex. Put your feet up. Sex, raise your ass. Sex, lie down and think about swimming sperm.

***Cut to Finding Nemo: Dory: Just keep swimming, just keep swimming* ** Sex. Sex. Sex. (Apologies again to my mother and my mother-in-law.)

I even bought one of those expensive ovulation kits where you pee on a stick every morning and it tells you when you are ovulating. One morning, I got the signal I was ovulating: ☺. No joke, that stupid smiley face told me I was ovulating and that it was a perfect time to have more sex and put my feet up. We waited; I never got my period, so naturally I thought I was pregnant.

I remember being at a Guster concert in Central Park. I was not drinking because I thought I was pregnant. Did I mention that? This whole time I was not drinking because I thought I was pregnant. I had two bachelorette parties that summer, and I did not drink. My friends thought the world was ending or I was dying from cancer.

Going back to the Guster concert, my husband and I were enjoying the show and I started feeling some rumblings in my lower stomach. I remember looking at him and telling him that I thought I was pregnant. He had the biggest smile on his face and held me. It was such an amazing, genuinely happy moment and it was all false. I was not pregnant at all. It turns out that I had gas.

What was happening to me? Why was I not getting my period? I started tracking my menstrual cycles using an app on my phone. *There's an app for that.* My cycles were completely irregular and that stupid fucking smiley face that told me I was ovulating was 100% wrong every single time.

Stop smiling at me asshole!

Around late October/November, I dragged my husband to my ob-gyn. I brought a calendar of when I had, or more accurately in my case, when I had not, received my periods. I thought this was normal.

It is probably just my body adjusting to being off the birth control, right?

No.

This was not normal. She started me on a low dose of Clomid. Nothing happened. I did not ovulate.

But that's okay, it was a low dose, I tried to convince myself.

Next month, she increased my dosage. Now it was December. Again, nothing happened.

All this time my best friend Shamecha was also trying to get pregnant again after her miscarriage. We had each other to lean on, to bitch to, and to support each other. It was great. Then on December 22nd, I got a call from my ob-gyn. She had left me a voicemail that said that I had PCOS, and that I should call her back, but that she was recommending me to see a **fertility doctor**.

Because I am a person of little to moderate intelligence I, of course, took to Google to figure out what the fuck is PCOS. It turns out that PCOS makes you **infertile**.

That was the word – **infertile**. That was the only word I could see, the only word that stood out to me. I lost my mind. I was hysterical. I called my husband sobbing and told him he had to come home right away. I was a wreck. I called Shamecha and we talked for a long time about what that meant. She was amazing, so supportive and perfect.

Four hours later, my husband actually walked through the door, which annoyed me, but I needed him so I let it slide. He reassured me that we would get through this and it would be all right.

We had no idea what "this" meant. Were there different levels of severity? Would I never get pregnant? Should we just start looking into adoption? What the FUCK?

The next day at work I was better, calmer, well somewhat. That is a lie. I was still a total wreck, but I had to pretend to live life. I stopped by Shamecha's classroom because, even though I was going through a life crisis, I remembered that she was due to take a pregnancy test soon. We always knew when the other was ovulating – true friends.

She told me that her pregnancy test came back positive. She spent most of the night crying to her husband because she was so happy for herself, but also sad for me, and she did not know how to tell me. I was genuinely happy for her but it was also such a shock. I was infertile and my biggest support system was pregnant.

Fan-fucking-tastic.

I sent her a long email about how I was very sad for me, but very happy for her, which was all true. This pregnancy stuck and nine months later Shamecha and her husband welcomed their first baby into the world.

That Christmas break was hard for me. I called the fertility clinic and left a million messages. Apparently, they shut the laboratory down around Christmas so no one could help me right away. As soon as they were back open in January, I had an appointment.

They told me it was because I was "persistent," which is code for I annoyed the fuck out of them and they finally just gave me an appointment to shut me up.

CHAPTER 3

The Fertility Clinic

THE FIRST RULE OF THE FERTILITY CLINIC IS THAT YOU DO NOT TALK about the fertility clinic. The second rule of the fertility clinic is that you DO NOT TALK ABOUT THE FERTILITY CLINIC!

One would think that these rules, like *Fight Club*, would be posted somewhere in, or around, the clinic, but they are not. They are the unspoken rules that cloud fertility. Not only do you not talk about the fertility clinic, another rule is that there is no talking to other people inside the clinic. We will get to that.

In early January, my husband and I went to the fertility doctor together. He took our medical and family history. He explained to me what the heck PCOS was and gave us our options.

PCOS stands for Poly Cystic Ovarian Syndrome. It is kind of a good thing because it means I have a ton of eggs, like a farm's worth of eggs – think Costco. But, it is also bad, because that means that no one egg can grow, to become dominant, and then release, to float down the fallopian tube, and into the uterus to be fertilized by my husband's amazing, totally nothing wrong with them, sperm. (I actually wrote that sentence on my own, not solicited by him at all, you are welcome honey.)

Are we all remembering that bizarre talk in fifth grade and then later in high school biology? It took me a while too. *What? Ovaries? Tubes? Eggs? Sperm?*

PCOS also comes with some other fun symptoms like loss of hair on your head, but growth of hair on your face. (Shout out to Sue at European Wax Center for keeping that shit in check.)

The doctor gave me a pelvic exam, feet in stirrups, vagina feeling the fresh fertility clinic air on her lips. It turns out that my uterus is also tipped back, which is normal, but abnormal. He showed me my ovaries, which to me looked like cookies and cream ice cream. The black chunks of "cookie" were the cysts that were covering each ovary. It was **unreal**; all I could see were black chunks.

The doctor, who we will call Dr. Lombardo (that is not his name – that is the name of the pizza place down the street from me, but sure, just go with it), told me that I had three options.

Correction, he told us. *US.*

My husband was there too and had a voice in this too. But he and I both knew that after my emotional trauma of thinking I was never going to get pregnant, I was really the one calling the shots of which line of treatment we did first.

My options were the following: Clomid and just hump like bunnies at home, Clomid and IUI (Inter Uterine Insemination), or IVF (InVitro Fertilization).

Dr. Lombardo recommended either tier one or tier two. He did not think we needed to rush into IVF and neither did we. Therefore, it was either Clomid and intercourse, or Clomid and IUI.

My husband left it to me. I chose Clomid and IUI. Remember, I still think I am never going to get pregnant on my own, and that we are never going to have children.

Maybe that's why I went into teaching in the first place because my body knew that I was never going to have kids.

Seriously, if you are a woman, this is how crazy your head gets, when you go through this. If you are going through this right now, I am sure you are nodding your head, because you know I am right.

Infertility mind-fucks you and it is not cool.

I started on the Clomid right away. Since I was not ovulating, it did not matter when I started.

The following week my doctor scheduled me for an HSG (hysterosalpingogram) in the radiology department at the hospital. I scheduled it for first thing in the morning because I am a school teacher. We only get a certain number of sick and personal days and I did not want to take a whole day off. I was going to take a half-day. Dumb decision.

Cut to Pretty Woman: Julia Roberts' character in the fancy store talking to the sales clerk who would not sell to her the day before, "Big Mistake. Big. Huge."

The second pearl of wisdom I will bestow on you is: if you are having a HSG, take the whole freaking day off. You might not need it, but you will feel better you took it.

I arrived at the radiology department on time. I had followed all the directions for what to do prior to the procedure, except taking Advil. I did not think I would need it. I have a high pain tolerance, and Advil is for pussys. I changed my clothes in my little room, I don the provided hospital wraps and glorified paper towel drapes. I could hear Dr. Lombardo and another patient, who was getting what I can only imagine was the same thing done to her.

When she was finished, they let me into the room. I lay down on the massive cold metal table. There were x-ray machines all around. He gave me a sponge-like thing to squeeze if the pain got to be too much. That was when I realized that maybe I should have taken the Advil. *Shit.*

The nurse was holding my hand. Once again, and I say, "once again," because during fertility treatment you are constantly in this position, my legs were up and the doctor was neck-deep in my vag.

Yes please, everyone this is my vagina. Vagina, this is the entire freaking world, and their mother, and sister, and med student, and whoever else wants to take a trip down my va-jay-jay lane.

Dr. Lombardo inserted the tube into my vagina. Then, he started pushing in the dye. The dye is what they use to see your fallopian tubes. The dye shows up on the x-ray and tells them if you have any blockages. When he inserted the dye, I thought I was going to simultaneously scream and pass out. I had tremendous cramping and discomfort. He looked on the x-ray and saw no blockages. All done. I went to stand up and felt extremely dizzy.

I remember almost saying aloud "*I'm sorry for being such a pussy,*" but I substituted pussy for wimp, because I didn't think my esteemed fertility doctor would appreciate me dropping the pussy bomb at nine-thirty in the morning.

This **sucked**, and now I needed to go to work and teach first graders how to do word problems on a second grade level, while I felt like my uterus was about to have a unionized strike and walk out of my body.

I eventually got dressed and went outside. I was sitting outside of NYU Hospital, on a brick wall bench, on First Avenue, on a cold Thursday morning in January, crying. Crying because all of this fertility stuff was too much to handle. I tried to handle it with jokes, because that is what I do. I tried to handle it with strength. I tried to handle it with logic, but really just handling it at all, was plenty.

I cried, and cried. I called my sister and cried to her. I sat there for almost twenty minutes feeling the freezing cold of the bench seep through my clothes to my skin.

Did the procedure really hurt that badly, or was I simply overwhelmed by my new reality? I didn't know. I walked to Second Avenue, got in a taxi to take me down to my parking garage near where I lived, got in my car, smiled at my parking attendants, as I always do, and drove to school to teach. When I got home that evening, I put pajamas on, got in bed, spooned Brady, cried, and slept.

CHAPTER 4

Morning Monitoring

WE WERE STARTING THE FIRST IUI PROCESS. DR. LOMBARDO, AND his team of amazing nurses and staff, explained to me that I needed to take the Clomid on days three to seven of my period. Then on day ten of my cycle, I needed to go into the clinic for blood and an ultrasound. The ultrasound is the wand-looking thing that they shove up your vagina to see your uterus and your ovaries, and, if the medication is working, your follicles that are growing on your ovaries.

What do you mean I need to go to the clinic for blood and ultrasound before work? ***Before*** *work? I leave my apartment for work at seven in the morning, what could possibly be* ***before*** *that? Ok. I can do this. We can make this happen.*

John and I left the apartment at six-forty-five in the morning. We drove up First Avenue. He waited in the car, so that I did not have to pay for parking (keeping your minion waiting in the car is a New York City thing, eye roll). I went inside to be stuck with needles, and to have a wand shoved up my cooter.

On my first day of morning monitoring, I thought I would be the first person there. It was four minutes past seven in the morning, and even in the city that never sleeps, that is still really freaking early to be at a doctor's office.

I walked in and that was the moment I realized, *holy shit, **everyone is infertile***.

I was probably the eighth person in line. There was a computer to sign in. I took my seat in the waiting area. No talking, no smiling, no eye contact with the other patients – unspoken rule.

I was surprised to see what these other women looked like. No offense to the entire female gender, but I was expecting older women – older women who were career driven and did not decide to start families until later, or older women who maybe just found their mate later in life. Oh and lesbians! I was expecting to see, and make friends with, lesbians.

But this was different. There was **every type** of woman on the spectrum. There were girls that looked like me, with mediocre blow-dried hair, pants from the Gap, flats and large tote bags. I tried to smile at these women before I knew "The Rules." There were young girls that looked like they had jobs in fashion, or marketing, or something that did not involve helping children wipe their noses. There were older women. There were religiously conservative women with their pushy, overbearing husbands – no judgement. There were lesbians, but not as many as I expected. I also tried to smile/make eye contact with them, but no-go.

In the order in which you signed in on the computer, they call you back to "The Blood Room." They actually call it that. "The Blood Room." This is where the nicest, friendliest, and most awake people are in all of Manhattan.

They ask you the same questions every time – name, date of birth, etc. Then, they take one vial of your blood quicker than you can even feel that your shirtsleeve is rolled up. They are amazing. Afterwards, they put you into a regular ob-gyn looking room. I undress just from the waist down, hop onto the table, and, once again, put those feet in the stirrups.

Say hello vagina! Don't be shy vagina.

The doctor comes into the room, asks me some bedside manner questions, and pretends to actually be listening to the answers, even though he/she is not. They look at my chart and before I can say, "Hi, I'm Karen," they have a lubricated wand so far up my cooter that I am pretty sure I can taste last night's sushi dinner again. *Mmm spicy tuna roll?*

They first leave the wand in the middle and press buttons on the ultrasound machine. (I later learned that they are measuring my uterine lining at this time.) Then, sometimes with warning, but mostly without warning, they shove the wand to the right, so much so that I almost fall off the table in that direction. I hold onto that faux leather cushioning *(what material is that?)*, and pray to God that I do not fall off the exam table while the doctor has his/her hand attached to the wand that is practically knocking me over.

They look at that ovary, measure, and press buttons. Then WHOOSH. Over to the **other** side, and *oops,* almost off the table I go. I give a little smile like, *It's okay, I didn't need that ovary anyway. You're the fertility doctor right? You can get me pregnant without the one ovary that you just bludgeoned out of my body right?*

They smile back and say slowly, "some light pressure."

Light pressure? The tip of the wand that you inserted into my vaginal canal is practically touching my hip bone. MY HIP BONE. Think about it people, that is like some crazy Cirque Du Soleil shit. Not really my idea of "light pressure."

So, I smile back, as I hold on for dear life and stare at the ceiling while taking deep breaths as if I am in Lamaze class.

Wait, if this is just morning monitoring, what is actual childbirth going to be like?

"All set," says the doctor as he/she takes off the sanitary condom of the wand that was just inside me, and throws it in the trash.

As I look at the ultrasound wand, I think it looks like it could be used for pleasure. So why was this experience so **not pleasurable**? The doctor tells me to wait for the phone call from the nurses, and they will tell me what to do. Once the blood results come in for the day, they take the information from my blood and from my ultrasound, and determine what my plan is for the next few days – "The Call."

"The Call" normally came anytime between the busiest part of my day and the "Are you freaking kidding me right now that I have to take this call?" part of the day. "The Call" never came when I was sitting, eating a sandwich, alone, at my desk. Never. For me, "The Call" came between one and three o'clock in the afternoon.

I nod to acknowledge that yes, indeed, I will wait for "The Call." *It is not as if I am about to hop on a plane to Bora Bora.*

I stand up, and, with the blue cloth that was just "covering" me, I wipe away the abundance of lube, like an eighteenth century whore, if eighteenth century whores were allowed lube.

Seriously, now I'm starting to feel badly for eighteenth century whores.

Why they give you that blue cloth anyway, I really do not know. I am naked and you are down there chillin' like a villain with my vagina. Why are we covering it up? Is it to depersonalize the vagina?

"So, if we put this blue drape between the woman's torso and her vagina, then we will just see the vagina," said "a man," somewhere. "We won't see the woman that we're talking to and smiling awkwardly at."

I truly do not get it. I put my clothes back on, head to billing, and check out. At which time, I exit the clinic through the waiting room and, of course, further check out all the females there.

Crazy! It's ***everyone.***

I go downstairs to my husband in the car waiting for me. I drive up First Avenue to the United Nations building. I drop him off there, so he can walk to work. He does not work at the U.N. That would be cool. His job is not cool. I continue onto the FDR to get to my school in Westchester. This was morning monitoring. In January, this was the process on days eleven, thirteen, and fourteen of my cycle. Then the insemination. Once my blood was "looking good," meaning my follicles were of the right size, anywhere from 17-20mm, the doctors told me I would be inseminated the next day.

If you do not know anything about fertility, an insemination is not what you think. I thought artificial insemination when I first heard it, but no, that is for lesbians. Essentially, they take my husband's perfectly working sperm, you are welcome again honey, and they shoot it up inside of me with a glorified turkey baster. I am sure there is a medical term for what that turkey baster is called. But as the disclaimers on the front, back, and subliminally watermarked, on every tenth page of this book, or whatever this pipe dream is that I am writing, while my kid is in in her jumparoo, and I am on maternity leave, enjoying life in yoga pants, will tell you; I'm not a doctor, so glorified turkey baster it is.[1]

When we first met with Dr. Lombardo, he explained the IUI process to us. He told us that once my eggs were ready, which was determined through the morning monitoring and blood results process, he would give me a trigger shot that would release my eggs, which were now the right size for ovulation, down the fallopian tubes. The next day, John would go to the clinic, and "give his donation." "Give his donation," is the medical term for – jerk off into a cup.

Dr. Lombardo then explained that my husband's sperm would go to the laboratory on site. There, they would clean it and buff it. He actually used the word buff, which naturally made John and me picture little Umpa-Lumpas with white gloves buffing each individual sperm. I have been told that is not exactly how it is done, but that is still what I picture. Then they take his clean, shiny, new car-smelling sperm, and shoot it up inside of me with the turkey baster. And maybe, just maybe, one sperm meets with one of my newly resized, remodeled eggs, and we make a baby!

Or, maybe not. Our first IUI had negative results. No pregnancy. No baby. I drank a bottle of wine that night, a bottle, and cried. John told me not to respond like that, but I did not know what other way to respond. I did the HSG. I did the monitoring. I did not drink. I watched what I ate. No luck. I allowed myself one night of wallowing. Back to the drawing board.

---

[1] Let it be known that I wear yoga pants because they are comfortable, and they do not give me a muffin top. I do not actually "practice" yoga. I also just wanted to add a footnote so it seems like I am writing something of substance, which I know, I am not.

CHAPTER 5

~

Second IUI

WE DECIDED TO DO ANOTHER IUI (INSEMINATION) THE FOLLOWING month. My doctor told me it might take many IUIs, you never know. It is now February 2012. My sister is still pregnant. She is due in the middle of March. I have been going in for the morning monitoring fun times as described previously, same as last month. My IUI is scheduled for tomorrow, Friday, February 10, 2012. I have already arranged to take the day off, due to the procedure. My phone rings at four o'clock in the morning; it is my sister, Katie.

"What's wrong? Are you in labor?" I ask, thinking there is no way the answer is yes, because she is not due for another five weeks.

"Umm… yeah, I am. We're at the hospital and I'm in labor," she said.

"Holy shit! Okay. Ummmm… I'm having an IUI today, but I will get on a plane as soon as I can," I say.

Katie lives in Chicago. I hung up and immediately started sobbing. This was too much to handle. My sister was having her baby early, and I am scheduled for an IUI because I cannot have babies at all. I am breaking down.

I pull my shit together, quickly call my fertility clinic, and start looking up flight information. I also ask my husband to Google if I am "allowed" to fly after an IUI. I decide that I do not care what the answer is. I book my flight to Chicago to leave a few hours after my IUI that same day.

My husband goes to the clinic in the morning and gives his "donation." I go in the afternoon, and get turkey basted. *That's right, I made it a verb.*

As soon as I am done with the IUI, I walk out of the clinic, hail a taxi, and head to LaGuardia Airport to get on a plane to see Katie. The whole day I receive constant text message updates about her labor from my brother-in-law.

I sit at the gate at the airport, crying hysterically, getting text updates. Then, I sit on the airplane, crying. We back out of the gate. All cell phones are supposed to be powered down, but I whisper on the phone to my brother-in-law because my sister just gave birth to the first child in our family. *Yay!*

I am bawling hysterically on the plane – the really attractive type of bawling, where the snot is gushing from my nose, and my face is red and puffy. People around me are pretending not to notice, while at the same time staring at me with their side-eyes.

Fuck you assholes! I just missed the birth of my first nephew because I can't get pregnant on my own, and I had to be turkey basted today! (Verb.)

I arrive at O'Hare Airport and push my way off the plane as only a true New Yorker can. I run through the airport, which is impressive since I have not run anywhere since high school field hockey practice in the fall of 1999. I make it to the taxi line and realize quickly that saying, "my sister just had a baby," does not make other people want to let you go in front of them.

I wait. Dying inside. Anxious, my heart is beating out of my chest. Almost in tears again, I wait. I take a taxi straight to the hospital, which is more like a nice hotel, but, sure, we will call it a hospital. I run (again, still impressed with the amount of running I am doing) to her room. I arrive, and see my sister. We both burst into tears as we hug the way only sisters hug. I apologize profusely for missing the actual birth. I meet my nephew for the first time. I hold him in my arms, and I know that I will never forget that moment for the rest of my life. I was proud of my older sister, my best friend. She was such a champion, and she made it look so easy.

About thirty minutes later, I go to the bathroom down the hall, and have massive, explosive diarrhea. Massive. The type of diarrhea that makes you ecstatic that you are using a single-stall bathroom. Crazy day. This IUI definitely did not work, with the stress and anxiety, the running, and the diarrhea. I might as well just forget about the IUI this month and focus my energy, and my crazy thoughts, on next month's fertility treatment.

The next day I was at Katie's house, getting ready to have her come home –mopping the floors, going to the grocery store – when I got the phone call. It was my sister. I pick up and all I hear on the other end is sobbing. I start to freak out. I immediately begin to panic. *Did something happen to the baby?*

We are all in their kitchen – me, my parents, my brother-in-law's parents, my sister's stepchildren. Everyone is having regular, normal, loud conversation.

I start to scream into the phone, "Kate is the baby okay?! KATE IS THE BABY OKAY!?"

My heart is beating so hard that I feel like I am sprinting down Lake Shore Drive to get to her. I realize that I am out of breath, and I am not even moving. My mother, who often wins the award for the loudest voice, and the most oblivious to it, keeps talking. I scream, "Mom! SHUT UP!!"

Everyone stops, silent, and stares at me, sitting there, on the phone. No one in that room knew what was happening in that minute, including myself. We were all on edge, scared, nervous, and anticipatory. Are we about to hear the worst news a family could hear at this moment?

"Kate, is the baby okay!?" I am shaking, screaming. Kate is crying so violently that she cannot answer me.

Finally, she squeaks out, "He's okay."

CHAPTER 6

My Nephew Sucks at Breathing

I take a breath and realize I had not been breathing. I nod to everyone in the, now silent, kitchen to acknowledge that my nephew is all right. They breathe. Through tears, my sister is able to tell me that since my nephew was five weeks premature, he had to do what is called the "car seat test." They put him in his car seat and attached him to machines that monitored his breathing. If he stopped breathing, it means that he failed the car seat test. He failed. He was being transferred to the NICU. Once in the NICU, it would be a guaranteed two-day stay there, minimum. Carter, my nephew, was not coming home that weekend, but he was all right. Once my sister, brother-in-law, and nephew, had settled in to the NICU, we all drove to the hotel-hospital to see them.

Now that Carter was attached to the machines, it was clear that he was having issues breathing. Every few minutes he would stop breathing, his machines would beep, then he would resume regular breathing, and the machines would go back to normal. My sister was a wreck. She just gave birth to her first baby less than a day earlier, and now, instead of being in bed recovering, she was sitting up in a chair, watching her son stop breathing from time to time. We all rallied around her as much as we could.

I flew back home that Sunday night, and went back to work as normal. I did not sleep for a few nights because the nightmare of my sister calling me crying hysterically was still fresh in my mind and haunting me. All the "what-ifs" were haunting me.

Two weeks later, I had February vacation from school. I flew back out to spend the week with my sister. We woke up every morning, went to the NICU, sat there for hours, fed Carter, watched Carter, got angry at everyone else around Carter for just doing their jobs, and went home. Lather, rinse, repeat the next day.

I was turning thirty years old that weekend. We had previously decided that we were going to celebrate my birthday in Chicago that year because my sister was supposed to still be pregnant, and she would not be able to fly. It turns out it was good we planned that way, for no one could have planned that her premature baby would be hospitalized in the Prentice Hospital NICU.

Thursday, February 23, 2012 Katie and I were hanging out in the NICU. For some reason, I could not stop drinking water. So much so that my sister even mentioned something to me about why I was going so crazy for water?

"I dunno." I answered her.

That night we did what my sister and I do best. We ordered a ridiculous amount of sushi for two people and drank wine. I was supposed to take a pregnancy test, for my IUI, the next morning. I had packed some with me.

Katie asked me, "Do you want to take the test tonight?"

"No," I said, "it's just going to be negative again, and if it's negative, it can wait until the morning to be negative."

The next morning, I did the familiar ritual of peeing onto a stick. I expected the test to be negative; all the other tests that I had taken up to that point were negative. Those stupid single or double lines mess with your eyes like a 3-D image from the 1990s. I quickly realized that I am not mentally stable enough for the lined pregnancy tests, and I graduated to the more expensive, digital word test that clearly stated "pregnant" or "not pregnant." This test was different from all the others in the past. This test said, "Pregnant."

I ran upstairs to Katie, who was getting ready. She gave me more tests just to confirm. We waited for those to say pregnant too, and they did! Pregnant! We went back to the NICU and continued our daily schedule, with one difference. I was pregnant. My husband was 900 miles away, and I was pregnant. He was flying in the next morning, and I was bursting at the seams to tell him. I am a person who sucks at lying; I am simply not smart enough, or creative enough, to be a good liar. I needed to withhold this information from John until I saw him, in person, the next day.

My pregnancy went off without a hitch. Funny, I cannot get pregnant on my own, not at all, not even a little bit, but once I am pregnant, I am pregnant for as long as a person is medically permitted to be pregnant. My first daughter was born in November – five days after her due date.

CHAPTER 7

This Motherhood Shit is Fucking Hard

I AM RELUCTANT TO WRITE A CHAPTER ON MOTHERHOOD IN A BOOK about infertility because, let's cut the shit, who wants to hear about my woes of being a new mom when they themselves cannot get pregnant. That is annoying. However, I just Googled how many words a "real" book needs to have, and it is a **shit ton.** So chapter on motherhood, here we go. For those of you who are officially annoyed, I understand, please feel free to skip ahead. I would also like to preface this section by saying that my children are my world. I love them to pieces. Please do not call child services on me for being honest. Thank you.

This Motherhood Shit Is Fucking Hard!

My water broke with Zoe around four forty-five in the morning on Thursday, November 8, 2012. I was supposed to be admitted into the hospital that evening to be induced. Instead, my water broke at home, everywhere. So disgusting. It was bright yellow, which scared the shit out of me.

Yellow? When Charlotte from Sex and the City's *water broke on the sidewalk because she was mad at Big, she didn't mention that it was yellow.*

We went to the hospital. We entered the little triage room, where the hospital staff figure out if your water has actually broken, or if it is a false alarm. My water had broken. I was admitted. We went to my delivery room.

My biggest fear of childbirth was shitting on the delivery table. That was my biggest fear, not the fact that after childbirth I was going to be responsible for a freaking child, nope, shitting. I asked for an enema the second I was admitted. They obliged. It was fantastic; I would highly recommend an enema to anyone who asks. The nurses started a Pitocin IV, which is a medication that makes the contractions happen. The nurse explained to me that my water was yellow because my baby had pooped inside of me, and it was important to get her out, hence the Pitocin. Apparently, eating your own shit is frowned upon, even in the womb.

The contractions started, and, hours later, the epidural was administered, which I would also **highly** recommend – even more so than the enema – amazing. Labor was going smoothly, progressing nicely. Around five o'clock in the evening, the nurses, who are the most amazing people in the world and who run everything, decide that it is time for me to start pushing.

I pushed for an hour and a half, which I thought was normal. Maybe it is? I still do not really know. At six-thirty that night out popped Zoe! She was mucusy and having difficulty breathing, so the doctors took her over to the little baby bed with the lights. They were hitting her chest with a small rubber pillow to break up the mucus. When they gave her back to me she had calmed down. They placed my daughter on my chest. It was amazing.

Once my epidural wore off, they took Zoe to the nursery to do whatever it is they do there, and the nurse instructed me to stand up.

Gunshot Wound to the Vagina – The Shit No One Tells You

Once I got feeling back into my legs, it was time to get up and go to the bathroom. With the **extreme** assistance of the nurse, I stood up. The second I stood up, GUSH, blood everywhere!

What? What is this?

I do not do well with blood, definitely not **that** much blood. There was a trail of blood from the bed to the bathroom; it was all over the bathroom floor. Black was coming in from the corners of my vision, and my ears started to sound like I was underwater.

I am going to faint. Then it hit me. *I **can't** faint. I have a child. I need to feed a baby, and change a baby, and take care of a baby.*

I snapped myself out of my faint, and continued to apologize profusely to the nurse. She helped clean me and rolled me to the recovery room.

I could barely move.

No one told me this. Why didn't anyone tell me this?

Moving from the wheel chair to the bed was almost impossible. Moving from the bed to the bathroom took forever.

No one told me this?!?!

I was transferred to a room with another woman who had just pushed out a ten-pound baby. She was exhausted, and the nurses were letting her sleep. The nursery was taking care of her baby, except for the feedings. I had Zoe with me, and all she did was cry. Cry. Cry. All she wanted was to be held. I had read enough books to know that I was not supposed to hold her, and fall asleep because that is how babies die. I was so tired, all I wanted to do was sleep, but she just kept crying.

My poor "roommate" who just pushed out a ten-pound baby probably hates me right now. I thought to myself.

I felt so bad. Eventually, we sent Zoe to the nursery so I could sleep. A quick half hour later, a nurse wheeled my daughter back into my room. I awoke, startled, "How did she do?" I asked over my infant's incredibly loud screams.

"Not happy," said the nurse, and practically threw the baby into my arms.

Well, at least it's not just me that she cries with.

The next day was peppered with visitors from both sides of our family. My roommate had visitors too. Sharing a room with someone when both of you have just pushed children out of your vaginas is really one of the least fun things I can imagine. Sharing a bathroom is even worse.

Every time I went to the bathroom there was SO much blood. Gunshot wound to the vagina. Blood everywhere. Blood on the toilet seat. Blood on the floor. Blood in places I did not even think I had walked or touched. I did not want to gross out my "roommate," so I got on my hands and knees, and cleaned the floor and the seat every time I went to the bathroom.

This sucks.

The next night we got our own room, and so did my roommate.

Two days after we got home with Zoe, and all of our family had gone back to their homes, John and I sat down to dinner. Zoe was screaming, crying in the rock and play next to the dinner table. I went to sit down in my chair and immediately popped up, like a crazy post-partum jack in the box.

John looked at me. "What was that?" he asked.

"I can't sit down," I said, trying not to cry.

"What's going on?" he asked timidly, because he really does not want to know the answer.

"I think I'm healing. I think my vagina is healing and it's painful and tight, like a scab, kinda."

I go upstairs and against every doctor's recommendation, I steal my daughter's Aquaphor and start gobbing it onto my taint/grundle/happy bridge.

Ahhh, much better.

Being a first-time mom is a wonderful experience, if you are a normal selfless person. For me, a selfish asshole, it was a **major** jolt to my system. What do you mean I cannot drink wine, watch movies, and sleep as long as I want anymore? Those things are of paramount importance to me. Screw you baby for taking all of that away!

Zoe was very colicky, which is a nice way of saying she cried **all** the time. **All** the freaking time. I was breastfeeding, which at first I loved, but then I didn't. I felt a ridiculous amount of pressure from everyone to breastfeed. How is it acceptable for the women at the dry cleaners to ask me if I am breastfeeding, and then to tell me how important breastfeeding is? Why is it anyone's business but my own if I am sticking my tit in my kid's mouth or not?

Zoe cried and cried. We thought that it was stuff I was eating, so we cut out pretty much everything. First sushi – that was a bad night. Then vegetables, we were awake for hours. Then dairy. Then everything. By the end, I was on a diet of peanut butter and jelly sandwiches for breakfast, lunch, and dinner. I did not understand how my child was getting the nutrients she needed if I was only eating peanut butter and jelly, but everyone told me to stick with it, so I did.

I was miserable. Miserable. All she did was cry, and when she was not crying, I was waiting for her to cry. I would take the twenty-six minutes of no crying and run a quick errand. Random people would approach me on my errands and say things like, "Oh, what a blessing. God bless."

God bless. God bless? My vagina might never be the same again. I cannot eat or drink anything. I am beyond sleep deprived. I might never get my body back. God bless? This is freaking Guantanamo Bay and you are saying, "God Bless".

Fuck you!

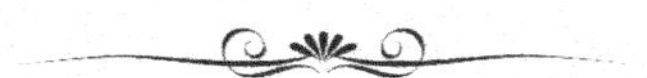

You know that saying "*It takes a village to raise a child*?" Well, it does not, and I did not asked for strangers to approach me and tell me how to raise mine. I needed to go to the supermarket. We needed everything. For whatever reason we were not able to go that weekend, so I decided to go with the baby. I had gone to the market many times before, but I had always picked up just enough stuff to fit into the bottom basket of my stroller, and nothing more. This time I needed a cart.

A cart.

How do I do this?

That is the question that every new mother asks herself, all the time. Things that used to seem so easy make you question, "How am I going to do this with the baby?"

I decided that the best way was to put Zoe in the baby carrier thing that strapped to my chest and get the cart. She was still too little to sit up in the cart, so this seemed like the best option.

It started out fine. Produce section – done. Chips and snacks – done. Around the cheese and dairy aisles she starts to freak the fuck out. She is burning up. She always runs a little warm, but she is on fire. Between my body heat and her body heat, and with both our heavy winter coats on, we are one huge radiator. She starts screaming-crying. I am used to it, but I start to realize that everyone around you stares at you when your baby cries. This is not going to end well. I hurry up and check out.

She is screaming. Burning. Screaming. I am turn red from embarrassment because people are staring at me and making stupid comments, like "Oh she's tired" or "She must be hungry." When I know, she just woke up from a nap, and had a bottle, and I, like the idiot I am, just decided to go to the supermarket. I take off her coat, again, because she is on fire. After paying for my groceries, I start to walk to my car. It is a little cold out, so I hang her coat over her head and wrap it around her without actually putting her back in it. She is still strapped to my chest in the BabyBjorn contraption, and still burning up.

I walk across the parking lot and a nice woman, in her car, lets me cross. *Thank you nice lady,* I think to myself. I continue to walk to my car. I notice the woman who just let me cross is circling around the parking lot and coming back in my direction, but I don't pay it any attention.

I put Zoe into the car, so I can load the groceries into the trunk and take my screaming child home. The woman in the car slows down as she drives past and says something to me.

"What was that?" I honestly could not hear her.

"You need to put a coat on that child!" She screams from her car rolling past.

"She's crying because she's too hot!" I scream back, unsure why I even feel the need to explain myself to this crazy cunt-bag in a Pontiac.

"You need to put that child in a coat!" She screams again.

That is it. I lose it.

"She's crying because she's too hot you fucking CUNT!" I scream.

"Nice! Really nice parenting," she yells. "Someone should call Child Services on you!" she screams as she drives away.

"ON ME?? ARE YOU FUCKING KIDDING ME?????!!!!!" I scream at the top of my lungs, as she drives away. My voice echoes throughout the parking lot. Zoe is still screaming. I throw all the groceries into my trunk and cry the whole way home.

Weeks later we receive the "go ahead" from my ob-gyn to have sex. I do not think I am ready, but I want to be "that wife" who has sex the first chance I can after having a baby. I want to, but I am scared.

We do it. It didn't hurt, but it didn't feel amazing either. Sex after childbirth is not the best sex of your life ladies. I hate to break it to you. But it does get back to normal, over time. I was still breastfeeding and, for me, having an orgasm while breastfeeding felt like I was reaching out for something, and I could almost touch it, but I could not quite get there.

When Zoe was around four or five months, I stopped breastfeeding, my body started to come back, and sex became great again.

The first four months of my maternity leave sucked. Don't get me wrong, I loved my baby. I loved her from the moment I knew about her in Chicago with my sister. I loved her, but I did not really **like** "it." Up until this point, I did not really like maternity leave.

Zoe was born in November, and I decided to take the rest of the year off. This was a very hard decision to make. I remember telling my husband, "Maybe we should get a trained professional to take care of Zoe, and I can go back to teaching because that's what I'm trained in, not this."

Having a baby born in November means that it was right in time for the weather to turn bad, and for me to be stuck indoors with a screaming child **forever**. John was folding the laundry one night and he said, "Honey, you don't have any socks."

I looked at him while breastfeeding Zoe. The exhausted misery look on my face was just permanent at this point, and I said, "I didn't go outside this week. You have to wear socks to go outside, that's why there are no socks."

He looked away and kept folding, scared to death that I was going to stab him in his sleep.

That January, I got a clogged milk duct that became infected (Mastitis). I had flu-like symptoms. I was freezing cold, but with a fever. Chills. My breast was sore and tender. It felt like someone shot me with a paintball gun when I was not wearing the official paintball padding.

That same week I also sprouted a new addition to my body, my first hemorrhoid. *Fun!* I was still breastfeeding and continuing to take my pre-natal vitamins, which made my shits extremely hard. It gave new meaning to the saying "ripped a new asshole" because my shits were actually ripping apart my asshole. I was taking a ton of Colace (an over the counter stool softener), enough Colace to make a two-hundred-fifty pound man pee out of his asshole. But not me. My shits were so hard they were tearing me up. Literally.

One night after breastfeeding Zoe, I went to the bathroom to poop. I don't know exactly what happened, but I remember feeling a **pop**. When I was done, I wiped myself. There was so much blood on the toilet paper that I thought my period started, but I knew it had not. Wrong hole. I looked in the toilet; blood was floating in the water. A lot of blood. *What the fuck?!*

John, my local hemorrhoid expert, was sleeping and had to go to work the next morning, so I tried my best to handle the situation. I put Zoe's pink plastic infant bathtub into my bathtub. I filled it with hot water. I got naked and tried to soak my ass in it. I was still about twenty-five pounds overweight and getting my wide ass into my child's baby bathtub was not an easy feat. I felt like Will Ferrell in *Elf*, when he is too big for the North Pole shower. My ass could barely fit low enough into the baby tub to touch the hot water. When I finally did finagle my larger-than-life ass into the tub, I could not get it out. I was stuck.

My ass was stuck in the baby bathtub inside my bathtub. I started to panic. Flail. Water was going everywhere.

What do I do? Do I call out for John to help me? Will our marriage survive this incident? Once he sees me soaking my hemorrhoid ridden ass in the baby's bathtub that I am now stuck in, he cannot un-see that.

I decided to try harder to get out. Eventually, and ever so gracefully, I made my way out of the stronghold the plastic tub had over me. *Success! I'm free!* I went back to bed and looked at the clock. Zoe will start to cry in about forty-five minutes for her next feeding. *Fan-fucking-tastic.*

I vividly remember waking up on the day Zoe turned four months old, getting into the shower and thinking: *I haven't slept, like really slept, for four months. This shit is intense; it's not like college with a week of finals and no sleeping. This is four months. This is a third of a year of my life that I am not sleeping. This shit is no joke!*

In addition to not sleeping, I also felt pressure to always look well-rested and somewhat put together, even though I was in between body sizes and exhausted. I doubled the amount of under eye concealer I used. I switched from my subtle brown mascara to blaring black and never switched back. I found it incredible how much makeup I could wear to make it look like I was not wearing any makeup at all.

I became an expert at sounding as if I was an expert. Family and friends would ask me normal questions about normal baby things, like feedings and sleeping, and I would answer them in my most direct authoritative tone. Then, I would sneak away to the bathroom with my cell phone and Google what the real answer was.

There was a feeling that I felt at the beginning of my maternity leave – was it boredom? Loneliness? I had completely lost what little bit of brainpower I had prior to having a baby. I also lost all social cues. I would sit on the play mat and play with the baby, lift one butt cheek, and just fart. All the time. I would burp aloud. All the time. Additionally, there is nothing like carrying your baby down the stairs and hearing the sound of spit up, **smack,** hit the hardwood flooring of the stairs that tells you, "this is actually your life, this is **it**." Getting back into society was going to be tricky.

Maternity leave gradually improved and I started to like my new position as my daughter's bitch. I often equate Motherhood to servitude. I am my baby's servant. I am my toddler's servant. I am my dog's servant.

"Make me a chicken nugget, servant!" said every toddler ever.

"Feed me, servant. Change me, servant. Stop my teeth from hurting me, servant," said every baby with their screams and cries.

**Cut to *Wedding Crashers* where Vince Vaughn's character is making balloon animals at the wedding.
Annoying child: Make me a bicycle clown!!
Vince Vaughn: Why are you yelling at me?
Annoying child: Do it funny man!!**

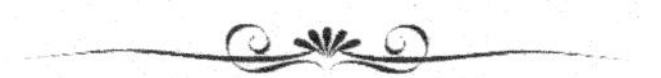

When my second daughter was born, (we'll get to that) I felt all the feelings I think I was "supposed" to feel when my first daughter was born. I was overwhelmed with joy, love, and the feeling of completeness. Because I am such a selfish individual, the adjustment from zero children (Brady excluded) to one child was the biggest shock to my life. The adjustment from one child to two children was significantly easier. I was already fully immersed in "mommy mode." It was like when my principal came to my classroom three days before the high stakes New York State tests, and told me that I was getting a new student who does not know a lick of English. At that point, what's one more?

Abby, my second daughter's, birth and recovery were significantly easier than Zoe's were. I think my body just knew how to bounce back because it had already been through that hell before.

Sex after Abby was a different story. We got the "go ahead" from the doctor. I was scared and still breastfeeding. We did it. Again, it did not hurt, but it did not feel good. It hurt more after the act, than during. What worried me was that my vagina felt huge. **HUGE**. It also had a terrible smell. It was a disaster. This was the text message that I sent to all of my friends. I am copying it word for word:

We just had sex for the first time. It was good.
Didn't hurt at all in the moment (hurts a little bit now),
But that's not the bad part.
My vagina is HUGE!!!!
HUUUUUUUUUGE!!!!!
huge huge huge.
Like throwing a hotdog down a hallway huge.
Like sailing a sailboat across the Atlantic huge.
Huge.
I'm so upset. I'm 33 years old with
Two kids and a fucking GINORMOUS vagina.
Basically my life is over.

The smell was like nothing I have ever smelled before. It smelled as if a wretched animal, like a raccoon or a skunk, had crawled up inside my ginormous vagina, farted, died, and was now decomposing. I called my doctor. I actually went into the doctor's office to have him swab my vagina to test for said rotting animal. The tests came back negative. The smell went away. After a few weeks, the sex started feeling normal again, good again, and then amazing again. My vagina was back to normal.

Thank fucking God.

CHAPTER 8

Time for Number Two

As my first daughter turned eighteen months old, I started thinking about having a second child. My husband and I definitely wanted two children. I wanted them around three years apart. All of my friends and family knew I conceived my first daughter, Zoe, with an IUI. I was always very vocal about it because I did not think there was any reason not to be. Many people told me that I would be surprised with how easily I got pregnant the second time.

"Your body will just 'know' what to do," they said.

However, I knew. I knew I would need fertility treatments, and I had a feeling I was going to need more intervention this time than I did with Zoe.

We started with Clomid around the end of June, the same dosage that I had been prescribed to conceive Zoe. Nothing happened. I did not even ovulate. We did what the doctors call "a step up" method. It was day fourteen of my cycle, and instead of waiting for a period that was never going to come because I was not ovulating, the doctors increased the dosage that same week and started me on more Clomid immediately.

Clomid. Clomid is a wonderful drug that has been around forever. My mother loves to tell me the story about how she was, "supposed to go on Clomid thirty-five years ago" when she was trying to get pregnant with my sister, "but then I went on a trip to London, and I found out I was pregnant." (The previous quote sounds better if you read it in that somewhat annoying, always condescending, "mom" voice.)

She tells me this story to be supportive, but, at the time, all I heard was, "Then I got pregnant on my own," which did not feel helpful while going through multiple fertility treatments.

Most people have great reactions to Clomid. Although, some women report having a thinner uterine lining on Clomid, in which case the doctors will see that during the wanding session, and they will prescribe a different medicine the following month.

I, however, became a binge eater on Clomid. Not like, *oh I'll take a little extra side of rice*, or maybe an extra snack here or there. No, we are talking BINGE eating. I would stand in the kitchen, and eat, and eat, and eat. I would eat until I felt sick, but I could not stop myself. All I wanted to do was eat my fucking face off. Clomid made me eat as if I was out of control. I sort of loved it because it was very out of character for me, and I totally hated it all at the same time.

I gained weight, which pissed me off, and made me start avoiding mirrors. All of these side effects would have been all right if I was not also going through fertility treatment, and, as I said earlier, the mind fuck insanity that fertility treatment causes.

So now, I'm chunky and infertile? Awesome.

We stepped-up the Clomid. I ovulated. We did an IUI. We traveled to Cape Cod to see our family for summer vacation. I started feeling all of those early pregnancy "symptoms": increased vaginal discharge, increased fatigue, and little twinges in, what I think, are my ovaries.

Wait two weeks, take pregnancy test (digital because we established that I am not sane enough for the line pregnancy tests), negative. Not pregnant, no symptoms, just the mind fuck.

It continued like that for four more months. My visits to the fertility clinic this time were different from last time. I, now, lived in the suburbs of New York City. My town is anywhere from forty-five minutes to three hours outside of the city, depending on traffic.

I would wake up at five o'clock in the morning, to leave the house at six o'clock, to get to the city and park my car, to be the first one waiting for the doors to open at the clinic. It was me and one other girl. We would wait in the elevator vestibule at six-forty-five every morning. She looked like me. I wanted to "make friends" with her. I even tried to forget about the unspoken fertility clinic rules and talk to her. It was a no-go; she was a strict rule follower apparently.

For four months, I did the morning monitoring – the early morning treks down to the city, the IUIs. I would leave the clinic, get on the FDR **again** and head north to work. I am teaching fourth grade now. By the time I got to my classroom it was anywhere between eight and eight-twenty in the morning. I felt like half of my day was done already, which in my mind made it totally acceptable to eat what I had packed for lunch that day. In reality, my day was just getting started. I would teach, pick up my daughter from daycare, be a mom, put her to bed, be a wife, go to sleep, and start the whole cycle again the next day. It was **exhausting**, mentally, physically, logistically, and emotionally.

After my second failed IUI, I asked my doctor if I could do the HSG again. That is the procedure where they shoot the dye up inside of me to see my fallopian tubes – the procedure that made me almost faint. I heard, through the underground fertility grape vine, that the HSG helps people get pregnant. There is no scientific proof to this, but women swear that they could not get pregnant, and then they did the HSG, and they got pregnant. People think the dye helps clean out the tubes and make things work better. I was willing to try anything. Therefore, I volunteered for another HSG.

Three years had passed since my first HSG, and apparently, the procedure was now in a different location. It was no longer at the NYU Hospital on First Avenue. It was around the beginning of the school year and I took the whole day off work because I was scared about having the same reaction to the HSG that I had the first time. I went to the new outpatient location on the Upper East Side. It looked like a regular doctor's office. When they called my name to go back I started panicking.

Why did I sign up for this? Am I a sadist?

I changed my clothes in the dressing room, and put on the robe/scrub-looking thing that they gave me. I walked into the room with the big machines. I climbed up onto the huge metal table, all the while explaining to every nurse that was around that I had a very bad reaction to this procedure last time, and that I might faint.

In walked the doctor. I was lying there on the table spread eagle, knees up, feet in stirrups.

Say hello vagina!

The doctor entered the room, and I explained how the last time I had the procedure done, I had a very bad reaction – a lot of pain, dizziness, etc. He understood. I also told him that my uterus is tipped back. I have learned in all of my years of fertility treatment that whenever I am in the stirrups, and someone is about to take a trip down my va-jay-jay lane, I need to tell them my uterus is tipped back. Otherwise, they get lost, and that can be painful for me when they are trying to find their way around.

I was lying there bracing myself for the pain, the torture, that I felt the first time. All I heard was, "all done."

That was it? Nice! I thought to myself.

I hopped off the table, got dressed, and did what any good employee would have done. I got sushi for lunch and headed home to rest on the couch until it was time to pick up my daughter from daycare.

I continued with more IUIs and more negative pregnancy tests. One morning during morning monitoring the sign in computer was down. Not working. I was the third person there. More women arrived. The stress level was through the roof. I thought we could all just do this on the honor system. I knew I was after the two girls ahead of me, who seemed as if they were friends and actually talked to each other, which was weird and unlawful. I knew who was after me. But people started to freak out. I looked around the room for the hidden cameras.

Clearly, this is a fun Steve Harvey social experiment?

But no. This was serious, and people were about to start pulling each other's hair out. Someone got a piece of paper and created a makeshift sign in sheet, to which people were practically elbowing each other just to get to.

Hello, ladies, honor system. It will be ok.

The DEFCON level of the clinic that morning intimidated me, but I secretly found it hilarious.

All of my negative IUIs those months were starting to affect me. I knew that I was going to get pregnant. I knew that I could carry a baby to term. I knew that it would all work out, and I tried hard to remind myself, "you have one child – you have one child." The issue with women, though, is that we want to be in control, we want to plan. I tried not be broken hearted every month because I had a child, but those months were rough.

After the fourth unsuccessful IUI, we decided to go forward with IVF. It was my choice and my husband supported me. Prior to starting IVF, I went back on birth control. This was for a couple of reasons: one reason was to schedule me into the elite IVF club at the clinic, and the other was to press the reset button on my ovaries.

Going back on birth control, even if only for a few weeks, was amazing. It was like pressing the pause button on the emotional drainage of infertility. I could drink. I could eat whatever I wanted. I could feel normal. I could stop binging for a few weeks. I could – breath.

CHAPTER 9

IVF for Dummies Class

THE WEEK BEFORE THANKSGIVING 2014, MY HUSBAND AND I attended our IVF orientation class. We both took half-days off of work. The calendar year was winding down and so was the IVF schedule at the clinic. Therefore, our class consisted of my husband and myself, and one other couple. Normally, there are many couples in the classes. We were told that we had lucked out, and soon I found out why. I assumed that IVF orientation class was all about the injections. The shots. I thought we would learn how to administer the shots. Were we going to practice on ourselves, or on mannequins? I didn't know, but I knew it was all about the shots. I told my friends, "This class is to teach me about the shots."

No. Wrong. Not even close.

Prior to the class I called one of the few people I knew who had gone through IVF, a former co-worker. She was wonderful. She took the time and explained everything to me over the phone, despite the fact that she just had a newborn baby at home and I am sure was exhausted.

She explained to me that the shots depended on what my protocol was. The protocol depends on what is wrong with me. She explained to me that there are stomach shots and ass shots. After talking with her, I felt confident I could administer the stomach shots, but I was nervous about the ass shots. I wasn't sure if I could reach the proper place in my ass to administer the shot, and my husband works long hours and is not home every night to shoot me in the ass. I went into IVF orientation class with lots of ass shot questions. Silly me.

IVF orientation class is like high school biology. There is a one hundred slide PowerPoint that explains exactly what IVF is, what it does, where the science originated, and how it has improved over the years.

The other couple seemed very nice. They were strict fertility clinic rule followers in the beginning. I tried so hard.

"Hi! I'm Karen. I have PCOS." No talking. No smiling.

What about a side smile? Nope. Just watch the slides.

"Where are the slides about the ass shots?" I whispered to my husband.

He looked at me like a stranger was talking to him, in the Quiet Car®, on the train. "Shut up and pay attention," he whispered back.

The slides continued. No exercise of any kind.

Ehh that's ok, that doesn't really apply to me.

No drinking alcohol of any kind.

Wait what? Like not at all?

Once the presentation was complete, we had many questions. What I quickly realized was that everyone does IVF for different reasons. I was there because I do not ovulate and I have too many eggs. Someone else might not make eggs at all. Someone might make eggs, but they are not genetically sound. Both us and the other couple had questions that were very specific to our particular infertility situation. Now, I realized why it was good that there were only two couples. Imagine doing this presentation with eight couples? Eight different infertility scenarios.

We received folders. They told us to focus on the legal documents first and the protocol papers second. The legal documents were daunting, my husband is a lawyer and they were still daunting.

What happens to your embryos in the unlikely event of both you and your spouse dying? What happens to your embryos if you divorce? Do you want to donate your embryos to science to help teach other doctors how to become embryologists? Do you want to donate your fertilized embryos to the world, so that one day I could be walking down the street and see a lovely couple (in my mind gay but they could be straight too) with a child that is actually my child - my egg and my husband's sperm? We had to make all of these decisions sitting at a conference table across from another couple, who was also making the same decisions.

Awkward.

Now came the time to talk about my protocol. They prescribed Follistim (stomach injection), with the possibility of adding Menopur (stomach injection). Both of these injections were to stimulate the ovaries to make the eggs— also known on the street as "stims."

Then, they prescribed Ganirelix (stomach injection). The Ganirelix was to suppress my body so that my eggs did not release on their own. We needed the eggs to release when the doctors were ready to catch them, and not a moment sooner.

"Omaha! Omaha! Hut!" (That's a Peyton Manning reference for the three men who are still reading this book. And no, I didn't forget that in the beginning I said there were five men and now I'm saying there are three. I'm saying there are three now because I'm assuming that my male readers are dropping like flies. *There's something about reading about this woman with an ultrasound wand up her cooter that makes me want to reach for my fantasy football magazine* – says every man **ever**.)

They told me that all of my injections, and syringes, were called into my mail away pharmacy for me. This is not the type of stuff you can pick up at your local CVS. They gave me the number for the mail away pharmacy. I learned quickly that I was on the phone with the mail away pharmacy more than anyone else in my life for that month. The number was saved in my phone, just a step away from being added to my favorites and labeled with a cute picture that would show up on my caller ID.

What about the ass shots? What are the ass shots? Why is no one talking to me about the fucking ass shots?

The other couple started smiling, a little, when I said "ass shots," and because I am an insecure person who measures my self-worth on if I make other people laugh, I continued to say it, a LOT. Maybe they are rule breakers after all? *Rebels.*

The ass shots are only after they take the eggs out of you, I was told. The ass shots are Progesterone in oil. The needle is huge, and the liquid is very thick. The nurse told us that we should hold the vial of the liquid in our armpits for a few minutes prior to injecting it in order to make the solution easier to inject. She then took out a mannequin from a secret cabinet in the wall. She took out some needles and a vial of the ass shot liquid.

Finally! Injection teaching time!

She nervously looked outside the conference room. She told us that she is not supposed to teach us this, but she would show us it, very quickly.

She "drew up" the needle with the progesterone solution and allowed my husband, and the other husband there, to inject the needle into the mannequin's ass so that they could feel the thickness of the liquid. That way, they would know how hard they need to push it into our asses. ("Drew up" is cool nurse talk for holding the vial of liquid upside down and pulling out the plunger on the syringe to fill the syringe with the liquid.) Then she took the mannequin away and hid it.

That was it? What about all the other injections? Who's going to teach me how to do this? What if I can't give myself the injections?

I asked all of these questions. The nurse seemed to have full confidence that I could do it on my own. She told me to download an app, *there's an app for that,* called Freedom Pharmacy. It has different videos of all the injections – how to prep them, how to inject them, where to inject them.

That night, I downloaded the app and watched in horror. The first video I watched was for the Follistim injection. There was a woman's voice on the video, and a woman's hands prepping the injection. She had very fake acrylic nails, and all I could think was, *"Really? You couldn't have found someone to be the hand model and injector with better nails?"*

I was fixated on the nails. The Follistim injection seemed pretty easy according to the nail-lady. It was a pen-like system. You dial out the knob to your prescribed dosage, pinch your skin, inject the needle into your skin, release the pinch, push the solution down into your skin, and pull out the needle. Nail-lady made it look very easy.

The next video I watched was for the Ganirelix, which was my suppressant so that my eggs did not release on their own. Nail-lady was back again – same nails, different colored t-shirt. This injection seemed pretty easy as well. Small micro-needle. It was not a pen system this time but an actual needle with syringe. I watched the video.

I can totally handle this and with a better manicure.

The next video I watched was the Progesterone in oil video. The ass shots. Same nail-lady. The prep looked like the others – easy.

I can totally do this. I'm a pro and all I've done so far is watch the videos.

The needle on this shot is significantly larger, and longer, than the others. The nail-lady prepares her ass for the injection. She pinches her butt and then FUCKING JAMS the needle in. I scream aloud in shock. I start to breathe heavy. My face turns red with anxiety.

What was that? Why did she jam it in so hard? What?

I rewind and watch the nail-lady bludgeon herself in the ass again.

Enough of this, I'm getting a glass of wine or two while I still can.

I put my phone down and try not to think about the trauma I just saw, while at the same time obsessing over it.

The next day, I brought my phone to Shamecha to show her the ass shot video. She yelps as the nail-lady slams the needle into her ass. Shamecha hands me back the phone, shaking her head.

This is going to suck.

We do our regular marathon Thanksgiving. I feel like there is a black cloud over my head because I know in just two days I am starting IVF.

December 1, 2014 is day two of my cycle. I wake up at four-forty-five in the morning. I leave the house at six. At this hour of the morning, the trip to NYC should take forty to forty-five minutes maximum. I am cruising down the highways in the black of the early winter morning, and everything comes to a halt. There is a massive traffic jam on the Deegan. I am stuck. I cannot go anywhere. I start to freak out as the minutes tick by.

Every minute that I am stuck in traffic is a minute that I am not early for the clinic. If I am not early for the clinic, I cannot get my blood and ultrasound first, and if I cannot get those things first, then I will not make it to work on time.

To most people getting to work on time is a relative thing. When you are a schoolteacher, you are contractually obligated to be in your classroom at a certain time. If you are late, everyone notices - not just because the other teachers are nosey bitches, but also because you have twenty-four ten year olds unsupervised outside your classroom. It is not okay to be late. It is a big deal – one that I take very seriously.

I am stuck in my car. My heart is pounding. I cannot even call my school to tell them that I will most likely be late because it is still too early in the morning. I punch the clinic's address into my GPS, praying that there is another way. I get off the highway around Yankee stadium. I drive on all the back roads like a mad taxi driver, swerving between lanes, running yellow lights (*okay, they were red, but whatever*). I am actually impressed with my driving, and, because I am me, I start to think that I am driving like Jason Bourne. *Awesome.*

The clock hits seven and I start to call my school because the early secretary should be there by now. I call repeatedly; she finally answers. I explain to her that I was in a ton of traffic, and that I am not even at the clinic yet. She seems surprised that I am talking so openly about the fertility clinic. I can tell she is surprised because when she repeats the words, *fertility clinic,* she stutters a little bit.

It's okay Rose. It's a fertility clinic, not a prison.

She tells me to keep her updated and that, if need be, someone will watch my twenty-four fourth graders until I get there.

No shit, you won't just leave them unattended in the hallway? Thanks.

Finally, I get to the clinic after it has already opened. It is roughly seven-twenty, which might as well be ten o'clock with the masses of people there. I know this is not going to go well, but I sign in and wait. I sit down and try to breathe, but my heart is pounding so fast that I am having a hard time catching my breath.

They call me, and a few other women, back to The Blood Room. I am still trying to catch my breath. We stand in the order that we were called, another unspoken fertility clinic rule. I wait for the nurse to call my name and tell me to take a seat. Standard practice. As I stand there, being respectful, a woman behind me says, "you can go," and she tries pushing past me.

I turn to her and in my nicest, bitchy-est voice say, "I'm waiting for her to call me. I'm being respectful."

Suddenly, the cunt cuts past me, and sits down in one of the chairs in The Blood Room.

This is NOT how the well-oiled machine of the fertility clinic works you asshole.

I start to lose my mind. I want to scream at the top of my lungs, but, like the sane person I am pretending to be, I simply sit down and give her a bitchy look. The blood nurses come in, and start taking our blood in the same order that we were originally called from the waiting room. In a series of very predictable events, however, the cunt that was behind me in line gets her blood taken first!

I know we are all women trying to get pregnant, and I should be nicer and more sensitive, but I **hate** cutters, and cutters at the fertility clinic are the **worst**. I take deep breaths, trying not to turn into the homicidal Hulk version of myself that I feel boiling on the inside. Finally, a nurse comes to take my blood.

"If that other girl was called after me, why did she get her blood taken first?" I asked, very calmly.

Now, the cutter is in the room, getting wanded up the cooter, and I am still in The Blood Room. The nurse apologizes and explains to me that because I am now an "IVF patient," a certain type of nurse needs to take my blood, not just anyone. She takes my blood, and sends me to get wanded.

I rush to school, driving like Jason Bourne the whole way.

I am so impressed with myself.

I get to work around eight-twenty, which is not actually humanly possible, but I did it. Rose is even surprised, which is huge because **nothing** surprises Rose. That day, I ask to see my assistant principal. She needs to know what is going on, especially after my almost-late, but totally on-time, moment this morning. December is a very busy month. I have forty parent-teacher conferences already scheduled for the middle of the month. Alone, that would be totally fine, if not for the IVF follicle extraction that is also pending for day fourteen of my cycle – the middle of the month. There is no way to know on December 1st what day the doctors will take out my follicles, so we will need to play it by ear.

Teachers are planners. We are not good at "playing it by ear." I explain to her that I am going through IVF. I explain to her what that exactly means, while simultaneously judging her for not already knowing.

It is 2014 right?

I ask for permission, if it comes to it, "May I please do my parent-teacher conferences over the phone?"

She agrees and tells me, "We just need to wait and see what happens."

No! We need to plan. We need a backup plan.

I get "The Call" later that day. It is time to start the shots.

CHAPTER 10

Shots, Shots, Shots

THAT NIGHT, I WAS INSTRUCTED TO START THE FOLLISTIM INJECtions. I already had all of my materials delivered to me. I organized and set everything up on my kitchen counter. After I put my toddler to bed, I start prepping the injection. I watch the video again, pausing every few minutes as I progress through each step. I am still not certain I will be able to give myself an injection at all, but I am trying to be strong. I am pretending to myself that I can do this, even though, deep down, I do not know if I can.

Worst-case scenario I could run up the block to a girl who I met at a drunken block party, who I vaguely remember saying she was a nurse. That was it! That was my backup plan in case I could not inject myself – run to a relative stranger's house and knock on their door. This was a completely new level of **not** normal.

I dial out the Follistim, pinch my stomach, and inject. I DID IT! I actually did it. I did not cry or pass out. I CAN DO THIS!! I start self-aggrandizing.

"I'm basically a nurse practitioner." I tell my husband.

He gives me an, *I'm not buying it,* look.

It was much like the look he gave me after I snuck into my kid's room to change the smoke detector battery, in the middle of the night, without waking her, and afterward I told everyone that I was essentially bomb technician that Jeremy Renner plays in *The Hurt Locker*.

Ok, I did one shot, big deal, but I was proud of myself.

Two days later, I go to the clinic again. This time, I leave my house at five-forty in the morning. No way was an accident on the Deegan going to make me late this time. And of course, because God has a messed up sense of humor, I am forty-five minutes early. I sit on the cold floor, in the elevator vestibule, waiting for the clinic to open.

Once you are an IVF patient you have reached the baller MVP world of the fertility clinic. In The Blood Room, you are practically a celebrity. All the nurses know your name.

Yes, like Cheers.

They all say, "hi," and ask you how you are doing. They also give you that sad half-smile, like they would for someone who just found out they only have weeks left to live.

I'm not dying people; I'm just trying to get pregnant.

They are very well-intentioned, I remind myself after each sorrowful death smile.

I get wanded, make my awkward small talk with the doctor, and head to school. I get "The Call" during the day. They are going to increase my Follistim dosage. I write down the directions, as I was told to do.

You should do that too; always write down your directions when the clinic calls you. You think that you're going to remember it, but when they call you at one o'clock in the afternoon and you're teaching or working, then going to daycare, then getting your toddler, then being a mom and wife all evening, and then you sit down to give yourself the injections, it seems like weeks have gone by since that afternoon call and it's very easy to forget.

I go home and do the injections.

This really isn't that bad. I can totally do this. It's fourteen days. I keep saying to myself, *I can do anything for fourteen days.* I find myself channeling my inner Cameron Diaz in *What Happens in Vegas*, when she states she "can do anything for six months." Too bad that my "anything" is IVF. Her "anything" is being married to Ashton Kutcher, not quite the same.

Two days later, I go back to the clinic. Super stardom in full effect. Blood Room. Wanded.

I got this shit down.

I get "The Call," which I have now imagined is the *Mission Impossible* lady with my mission **if** I choose to accept it. In the morning, the doctor says to me, "Okay, looks good. Wait for 'The Call.'"

I smile, "You mean my *Mission Impossible* mission if I choose to accept it?"

"What?" the doctor asks me with an incredibly confused look on his face.

"I like to think of 'The Call' as in *Mission Impossible.* This is my mission if I choose to accept it, which I do." I say with a smile of a seven-year-old kid on my face.

He stares at me blankly. He looks down at my medical chart, checking, I am sure, to see if I am taking uppers. He is shocked that someone going through IVF would look at it this way.

"Okay…sure. Wait for your mission call," he says. I know he is patronizing me, but I don't mind.

I am in the middle of small group instruction, when I get "The Call." My small group of students wait patiently; they are amazing. The nurse tells me I am not responding to the Follistim as they would have liked.

Bummer.

We need to add another injection. She already called it into my mail away pharmacy, and the pharmacy will be calling me shortly.

She explains that this medication will need to be mixed, and I should watch the video several times. She explains the ratio of how many powders to how many solutions, which I will be mixing. She assures me that this will all make sense once I actually administer the shot.

I am taking diligent notes, while also behavior managing the rest of the class who, naturally, think a phone call means they can behave like Armageddon arrived. As we are getting off the phone, she adds one last thing.

"Oh, and you should know that this injection will sting as it goes into you. You should know that, so when it does sting you don't think something is actually wrong." She says.

"Fantastic!" I say with a huge smile on my face. I cannot react the way I want to react because my students are right there.

"Did you hear what I said? It will be sore, it will sting, but that's normal," she adds because clearly my emphatic response was not socially appropriate.

"Yup, I heard you. Sounds great! I'm looking forward to it," I say energetically.

"Okay...,"she adds, "call us if you need anything, or have any questions about the mixing." She is worried; she thinks I did not get the message at all.

"Sounds great," I say, "Thank you!"

I receive the call from the mail away pharmacy minutes later. Again, my students patiently waiting. The new injection, Menopur, will arrive at my house that afternoon.

Damn they're fast. It's like Domino's Pizza delivery for IVF.

I get home and the Menopur arrives. I think about how much easier life would have been for those drug dealers on *The Wire* if they just had an efficient mail away pharmacy as I do. I put Zoe to bed.

I watch the video multiple times. The nail-lady is back. I watch her mix the powder and the solution with her acrylic nails.

Really? There wasn't anyone else, who saw these videos, who thought her nails are going to be distracting to some (okay, maybe just to one) questionably sane women going through IVF like myself?

The video tells me to inject the Menopur into my stomach. I get my Follistim ready because I was told to continue with the Follistim, and add the Menopur on top of that. I inject the Follistim into the left side of my belly button area.

I have the Menopur video up and ready, pausing every few minutes, while I am mixing my Menopur. I look at my kitchen counter.

Holy shit, I think to myself, *I've created a crack den! I live in a fucking crack den! This is NUTS!*

The nurse was right. I totally understand the mixing and I inject myself with the shot.

Yup, right again! It stings. Wow, that sucked.

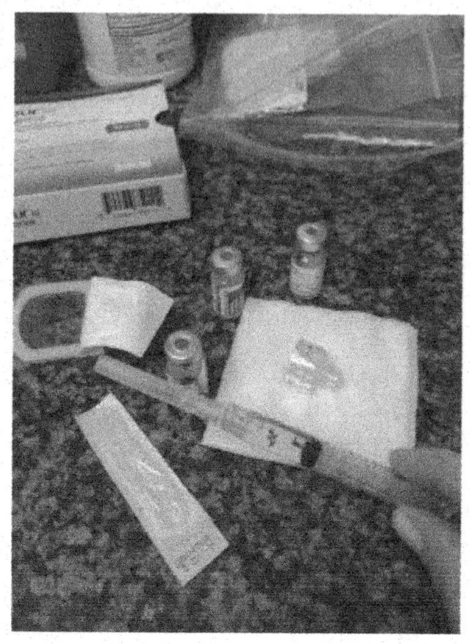

My Crack Den – notice the better manicure than the video nail-day

The next day my stomach is sensitive to the touch. I try to pick up my toddler but even the slightest touch sends me into excruciating pain. I cannot hold her. The pain brings tears to my eyes – partially because I am truly in that much pain, and partially because I want to be able to hold my toddler and not hear her cry and whine that she wants Mommy to carry her.

That night I open up my crack den promptly at eight o'clock as usual. I inject the easy one first, the Follistim. This time, it burns like crazy. Tears come to my eyes.

What the fuck? This was the easy injection. Why does this kill right now?

I start mixing my Menopur. I find myself taking deep breaths; I have the lights dimmed in the kitchen/crack den. Apparently dimming the lights is part of my routine now that I am deep into the IVF crack world.

I can't do it. I cannot inject this into me. It hurts. It's unnatural to want to inject yourself with something that you know is going to hurt you.

I try again, and again. I just can't do it. I walk out to my husband who is sitting on the couch.

"I can't do this. It's going to hurt. My stomach is so sensitive right now. The Follistim just killed me, and that's the easiest one."

"You can do this. This is nothing. It's fine," he says to me, clearly trying to tough-love the shit out of me.

I don't need Denzel Washington from Remember the Titans *right now, I need love and support.*

He holds my hand as I inject the Menopur needle into the right side of my belly button area.

Holy shit it burns!!

I start to sob, with the needle still in my hand. I cry so hard that I am shaking. John slowly, and carefully, takes the needle away from me, and puts it on the coffee table. It is in that moment that I feel like a true junky. I lean back on the couch like heroin addicts do after injecting themselves with their high.

Okay. I don't know any heroin addicts, but that is what Jesse and his girlfriend did, in Breaking Bad.

Except my leaning back after the injection is not in a high state of euphoria. It is quite the opposite. It is my low. It is the lowest I have been throughout this whole process. John does not really know what to do or how to handle me. I can tell that we have entered the no sudden movements' realm of the IVF process. I cry for a little longer and then get over myself. I clean up my crack den and go to sleep.

At the clinic the next morning, I tell them that the Menopur **sucks**. I explain that it made my stomach very sensitive, so much so that now the Follistim injection is painful, and Follistim is not typically a painful injection. The nurses understand and explain to me that I can move some of the shots down to my thighs. We make a plan to keep the Follistim in my stomach but to move the Menopur to my right thigh.

The doctor is wanding me. We can see the follicles growing.

Finally! Finally, they are growing because at first, nothing was happening.

"They seem to be responding to the Menopur," says the doctor.

Fan-fucking-tastic, I think to myself.

I continue on the Follistim and the Menopur for another day or so. Now that I have moved the Menopur down to the thigh, everything is better. It still stings at the injection site, but my stomach is better. The Follistim is not painful. I can carry my toddler.

Good. IVF isn't that bad. I can do this. We had a little blip on the radar with the addition of the Menopur, but I can totally handle this.

I am back to thinking that I can do anything for fourteen days.

Now, it is time to add my suppressant. If you remember from the IVF orientation class, the suppressant is to suppress my body, so that my body does not naturally release these follicles before the doctors are ready to grab them. The doctors tell me to start my Ganarelix in the mornings and to continue with the Follistim and the Menopur in the evenings. I am now up to three shots a day. Ganarelix, in the morning, in my left thigh. Follistim, in the evening, in my stomach, and Menopur, in the evening, in my right thigh.

It is now Wednesday, December 10, 2014. I have parent-teacher conferences all afternoon. Then, I have to rush down to the city for my husband's yearly stuffy, boring, but lovely, holiday party at the St. Regis. The whole time I am there, I am thinking about getting home to my crack den and doing my shots. I find it very distracting. I get a glass of wine just to hold, so that rumors of me being pregnant don't start flying around. That would really take the cake – people thinking I am pregnant because I am not drinking, when really I am not drinking because I cannot get pregnant.

I am not allowed to drink alcohol during the IVF process. At one point, by accident, I take a sip of wine. I just stand there, with it in my mouth like mouthwash; my lips pursed, my cheeks puffed out.

What do I do? I can't spit it out. Fuck! Oh well, down the hatch it goes.

I switch to water and do not make that mistake again. After the dinner, we rush home so that I can do my injections. I get up the next morning at the ass crack of dawn and go down to the clinic. At this point, I am going to the clinic every other day.

I get all my parent-teacher conferences done.

Success!

No IVF interference with that. This year, we are doing Christmas at my house on December 13th.

I didn't mention that? Yes, of course. I'm a working mom, going through IVF, forty parent-teacher conferences, and hosting Christmas dinner at my house. Totally do-able, said ***no one****.*

My sister, brother-in-law, and my two nephews *(yes, she has two now, she is very fertile)* are staying at my house. On Saturday morning, I head down to the clinic in the city. The doctors think I am getting close. I have roughly seventeen follicles or so, which is good. They want me to get ready to pick up an additional trigger shot. I already have an Ovidrel shot, at home, in my fridge, but I will need another trigger shot in addition to the Ovidrel. The doctor explains all of this to me while wanding (verb) my cooter.

She explains that there are two pharmacies in all of Manhattan that can make this additional Lupron trigger shot. I explain to her that we do not actually live in Manhattan, and that today is Christmas at my house.

"Oh, so not at all stressful," the doctor says sarcastically, which I, of course, utterly appreciate. She tells me to wait for the *Mission Impossible* phone call and they will tell me what to do. I drive home and start to prepare the dining room table, and the food, for Christmas dinner in a few hours.

"The Call" comes in. I will need to give myself the two trigger shots tonight at exactly ten o'clock. I am being scheduled for surgery, to take out all of my follicles, on Monday morning at nine-thirty. They give me the name of a pharmacy in Dobbs Ferry, about twenty minutes away from my house, that can make the shot. I call to make sure they have the Lupron in stock. I call the clinic back, and they call in the prescription for me. John drives to the pharmacy just in time because, of course, they are closing early on Saturday. I am still making Christmas dinner, and my toddler is playing with her two cousins. It is total chaos.

My parents arrive to celebrate Christmas with us. My father walks in with the worst attitude, because he is annoyed that we are not celebrating Christmas on actual Christmas Day. Within minutes of his arrival, and after multiple aggressively inappropriate comments on his part, I approach him and ask him what his deal is. My father, who is missing the sensitivity chip to his emotional control panel, explains to me that this has been really hard on him because my mother has been sick.

Really hard on him? Is he fucking kidding me right now? He's retired!!! The only thing he has scheduled to do on any given **week** *is go to Whole Foods. I'm sorry, are you a working mother of a toddler, undergoing IVF treatment, forty parent-teacher conferences and hosting Christmas at your house?!?!?!*

I wanted to take a running jump off the wall, land like a flying monkey onto his shoulders, and rip his head off. Instead, I managed to articulate something relatively sane like, "I know this has been hard on everyone, but it's for the children."

We get through Christmas presents and dinner. Aside from my nephew throwing up and having diarrhea everywhere, it turned out to be an all right time.

After my parents left, I began prepping my last crack den moment of 2014. I started about five minutes before ten o'clock because I wanted to get everything ready so I could inject exactly at ten. I inject both shots while my husband, sister, and brother-in-law are all hanging out in the family room, drinking. I walk into the family room and sit down. John pushes on my sweatshirt near my stomach.

"Why is your sweatshirt sticking out like that?" he says.

"That's not my sweatshirt," I tell him, "that's me; I'm so bloated from all these follicles in my ovaries that I'm busting out."

"Oh," he says, as he gives my brother-in-law a look like *oops*.

My brother-in-law laughs and gives John a look saying, *"Dude, you're a dead man – it was nice knowing you."*

CHAPTER 11

Retrieval - Taking Them Out

MONDAY MORNING, DECEMBER 15, 2014, WE DRIVE TO MY DAUGHTER's daycare to drop her off and head into the city for my egg retrieval. We leave the house at six-forty-five in the morning in order to get to daycare exactly at seven when they open. We did not want to take any chances with traffic and getting into the city during rush hour, especially because the whole IVF process would be shot to shit if I missed this surgery time window.

We pull up to daycare. There are Con Edison electric company trucks all over the road.

Weird, I think to myself.

We pull into the parking lot, and standing there, outside of her car, is the Director of the daycare.

"There's no power," she says, as I roll down my window. I am driving because I need to be in control. My husband understands, and is not contesting because he does actually value his life, even though he has told me multiple times that when I drive him around he feels emasculated.

"When is the power going to come back on?" I ask calmly, trying not to freak out.

"We have no idea; they are working on it now. I can't get inside. I can't even email the parents to tell them," she says. As she is talking, I am not really listening. I just look at her, wondering if she would judge me, if I just handed my child over to her, and told her I would pay her out of pocket to watch Zoe, and drove away. My conclusion – probably.

What are we going to do? I start thinking of friends and family in the area. Where could I just drop Zoe off so suddenly and unplanned? It has to be my parents, but they live twenty minutes north of where we are right now. The fertility clinic is south, and by going totally out of our way we are risking losing our surgery window, and therefore making this month of injections and hell all for nothing.

I make the decision quickly. It has to be my parents. I pull out of the parking lot and start speeding down the hill. We call them as we are heading there and explain that we are on our way to their house to drop Zoe off. I also explain that this is an emergency, and they need to be okay with it. They are, because they have no choice. Within minutes, we arrive at my parents' door (thanks, again, to my Jason Bourne-like driving skills). We literally bring Zoe into the house, leave her in the front hallway with my mother, and run back to the car.

I speed. I speed everywhere. I am shaking. This was not how this morning was supposed to go. We were early. We were going to be early.

We brought our Kindles with us because we were going to be so early that we were going to read in the waiting room. Now, I am scared that all those shots, all those injections, all those tears, were for nothing.

I am going to miss this. What happens then? I don't remember seeing the slide during the IVF class that explains what happens when life fucks with you and you miss your surgery window. I make a mental note to tell the doctors that they should add that slide.

As we are driving down the FDR, I begin to realize, that we are okay. We are making good time. The traffic could have been significantly worse, but we are doing all right.

We enter the clinic. It is a barren wasteland, pun intended. No morning monitor taking place. They shut down the laboratory at the end of the month. No people in sight.

This is weird.

We go to the second floor and wait in the waiting room. It is almost eerie how quiet the clinic is. John and I are not sure we are in the correct location. I feel as though maybe they forgot that I was supposed to have surgery this morning. Eventually, a nurse comes out to get us.

My husband and I are escorted into the back. I change, put on my scrubs, and lock everything in my locker. The nurse brings me to a small room where my husband is sitting. She starts taking my vitals. She gets out the blood pressure cuff, and, at that moment, I lose total control.

"My blood pressure might be slightly high right now because we've had a really tough morning already," I start to sob. Sob. The type of sobbing that makes you sound like you are gasping for air.

She looks at me like, *What the fuck?*

Even though she did not ask me any follow up questions about my hysteria, I continue talking, completely unsolicited.

"We went to drop my daughter off at daycare," I am sobbing in between the words, and she probably does not understand what I am saying, but, clearly, this woman is my confessional right now, so she goes with it.

"There was no power and we couldn't drop her off, so we had to drive to my parents' house, which is twenty minutes out of the way. We just dropped her there and ran, and she's probably really upset, but we made it; we made it here on time, but my blood pressure might be higher than normal because of that." Blaaaaah. Done. Diarrhea of the mouth, done. She does not engage in the conversation with me. She just keeps doing her job. The doctor comes into the room.

"Hi Karen, how are you?" she asks. Rhetorical! It is a rhetorical question, but I cannot handle normal social cues right now.

"I've had a rough morning," I say through tears, "there was no power at my daughter's daycare, and we were rushing, and I think I'm okay now, but it's been a rough morning."

She smiles, and looks at me as if to say, *Why are you telling me this? me this? Don't you know that "how are you" is a rhetorical question, especially at the fertility clinic?*

We move on. She explains that I am about to go into the surgery room. She tells me that I am going to walk into the room. I am going to climb up on the table, lie down, and get started with the anesthesiologist. I have my glasses on because contacts are not allowed. I ask her what is going to happen to my glasses during the surgery because clearly my mind is obsessing over the small things, to not think about the big thing. She explains that my glasses will be fine.

I tell her that I have a few questions for the doctor. We are traveling to Puerto Rico the following week with my sister, brother-in-law, two nephews, and step-niece and nephew. Following the procedure, I am supposed to start the ass shots. I am concerned about traveling with needles. Firstly, I would like a doctor's note stating that I have permission to travel with needles. Secondly, I would like to inquire about going on the progesterone suppositories, instead of the ass shots. I have heard through the IVF grapevine, that the suppositories are significantly easier, although messy. Thirdly, I remember in the IVF orientation class there was a slide about no swimming. I am going to Puerto Rico and I will be swimming with my toddler, and I need to know if this is allowed. I am not talking like Michael Phelps swimming; I am talking wading around in the kiddie pool. This doctor tells me not to worry about those questions now, and that we can ask my doctor all of those things after the surgery.

I say goodbye to my husband, who goes off to make his sperm donation, iPad in hand because he is a pro at this by now, and he does not care for the porn supplied by the clinic.

I walk into the surgery room and hop up onto the table. The anesthesiologist introduces himself to me, and, of course, I begin to tell him the story of the power outage and rushing Zoe to my parents' house.

Why? Why am I telling this man this? He doesn't care. I'm starting to get annoyed by the sound of my own voice, and yet I can't stop. I keep going and going.

He has injected all the needles, and intravenous lines, into my left arm. He has given me a local anesthetic, and is gearing up to knock me out. It is exactly nine-thirty.

Where is Dr. Lombardo? I thought that this shit was timed to the freaking minute? I did my trigger shots exactly at the minute, so that I don't mess up this surgery. Is it not exactly at the minute?

I, of course, ask this question.

"It is not down to the minute," says the nurse, "it is alright, there's a one to two minute window."

I keep looking at the clock. Finally, Dr. Lombardo walks in.

"Last, but certainly not the least." He says. He is referring to the fact that I am the last IVF patient of the year 2014. They are winding down their laboratory to re-calibrate the machines. I smile at him.

"I have two questions for you Doctor," I say.

"Oh, shhhhh, not now," he says, "now just go to sleep."

And I am out. The next thing I remember, I am on the gurney, being wheeled out of the room, and the first thing I say is, "Are we late?"

"Late?" asks the nurse.

"Are we late because the doctor was a little late?" I am sure my esteemed reproductive endocrinologist appreciates me telling him, in my twinkle dust state of consciousness, that I think he was late to his own surgery.

"No sweetie, you're done. The surgery is all done," says the nurse.

"My husband? Where's my husband? Can I see him?" I ask. You would think I was just pulled from the rubble of a collapsing building with the urgency of seeing my husband in my voice.

"You will be able to see him after recovery," someone says.

"My glasses? My glasses were on that other rolly thing," I say.

"Your glasses are right here," she says. I suddenly realize that I am on that rolly thing, and I did not even feel them move me.

Drugs are awesome.

"I still have two questions for the doctor," I say.

"Shhhh, time to rest and recover," says the nurse.

"How many eggs did you get?" I ask, clearly ignoring the rest/recover mandate.

"Thirty-three. They got thirty-three eggs," She tells me.

Holy shit!!! Thirty-three eggs!?!? Are you kidding me? That's like insane right? Damn. Thirty-three eggs, no wonder I was so bloated and huge, my ovaries were carrying thirty-three fucking eggs. Wow.

"Time to rest," they say as they roll me to a stop in the recovery room.

Yeah, alright, rest and recover, but I need to know if I can go swimming with my toddler. I don't really want to rest and recover. I want to get answers to my questions and get out of here. I can tell they're getting slightly annoyed with me because I'm not acting the way I'm supposed to. I feel totally fine. I feel awake, now.

I keep thinking about how the first thing out of my mouth when the anesthesia wore off was, "Are we going to be late?" Thank goodness, it was not something bad, or, knowing me, inappropriate. Then, I start thinking about what other people say the second they wake up, when they are still kind of dreaming. What types of messed up shit do these nurses and doctors hear all the time, and do not even acknowledge? I should ask them that question.

"Excuse me nurse?" I say. "I still have two questions for the doctor. I really need to talk to him."

She is annoyed. She asks me what the questions are. I explain them to her. She nods, and I know I have won. The doctor will be here soon.

Moments later, in walks Dr. Lombardo. "Hello, I hear you wanted to see me?"

"Yes, Doctor, I'm sorry to bother you, but I have two questions for you," I say.

"Do you remember telling me that you had two questions for me before the surgery?" he asks.

"Yes," I answer affirmatively. "I had two questions for you then, and I still have two questions for you now," I say.

"Wow. That's incredible. Your brain clearly works very well on drugs," he says emphatically.

I smile the biggest smile ever. He has no idea. I take this comment as single handedly the biggest compliment of my **life**. Later, I tell the story of how my doctor told me that my brain works well on drugs to all of my friends, and family, and quasi-strangers for the next three weeks. I even told the woman who does my manicures. I was elated.

Finally, I ask him the two questions. He begrudgingly tells me that I am allowed to swim, but that I need to take it easy. He agrees to put me on the progesterone suppositories, but he explains that they are very messy, and that if I am at the pool, wearing a bathing suit, it might be easier to just do the shots.

I feel successful. I got the approval to swim, and he is calling in the prescription for the suppositories. Now, I can make the choice if I want to do the ass shots or the suppositories. He also gives me a letter stating that I can travel with needles without the TSA doing a full cavity search up my asshole, which they will most likely do anyway because I am traveling with a toddler and clearly smuggling heroin in her food pouches.

Now, I can recover in peace. I wait less than thirty seconds.

"Nurse?" I say, "I think I'm good. I want to go now."

She explains to me that it is not that easy, that we need to take it slow.

Yeah, I get it, take it slow, but I have a toddler to get home to, and I feel totally fine, and I want to leave. I want to see my husband. Does she want me to explain the whole story about the power outage because I totally will, don't test me lady.

She sits me up in bed and makes me sit there with my feet dangling over the side for a few minutes.

"Nurse?" I say, "I think I'm good with this step."

She is annoyed. She comes back over. She helps me stand up.

I am good. I'm good. This is so annoying.

She brings me over to the bathroom. "You are not allowed to leave until you urinate," she says like a Navy Seal drill sergeant, "try now."

Damn lady, alright.

I try to go to the bathroom. Nothing. No pee. I walk outside and sit in the huge leather medical chair. It is so large, I feel like Lily Tomlin just had IVF surgery. She gets me apple juice. It tastes amazing. I drink it all.

Good. Now pee.

I go back into the bathroom. Nothing.

Mother Fucker! I just want to pee, so I can get the fuck out of here. I go back to my Lily Tomlin chair. There's another girl, who just got out of surgery too. She is in the bathroom. She's peeing! Lucky girl.

Later I ask the nurse what the other girl's surgery was, if I was the last IVF patient. "D&C," the nurse tells me, and my heart falls down to the pit of my stomach. I should not have asked. I feel horrible. The other patient pees successfully and leaves.

I take a moment to think about this whole process. They are trying to put life into me, by taking out my eggs, and this poor girl had life growing inside of her and for whatever reason, usually and often for a miscarriage, they needed to suck it out with a glorified Dyson. It is heartbreaking, all of it.

After trying to go to the bathroom, four times, the nurse tells me to take a cup of warm water and to pour it down my puss, and that will help me pee.

Why didn't you tell me that fifteen minutes ago??

I take her advice. It works. Fantastic. I can go now. I get dressed and meet up with my husband.

"How do you feel?" he asks me.

"I feel fine, totally fine. They got thirty-three eggs," I tell him.

"Wow, that's a lot right?" he asks.

"Yes honey, that's a lot."

He drives me home. I go up to bed. He drives up to my parents' house to pick up Zoe and brings her back home. We wanted to get her before it was her naptime, so she could nap at our home, and not there. I spend all day in bed. It was somewhat amazing. It is sad that a working mother has to go through IVF treatment to get one day uninterrupted in bed, but I will take it.

After the IVF retrieval procedure, there were many symptoms I was not ready for. All these symptoms were outlined in the IVF orientation class slide show, but I was still taken by surprise. When you have as many follicles as I had, you run a risk of experiencing something called Overhyperstimulation, which means your ovaries are swollen as fuck. If this happens to you, then you cannot put the fresh embryo back inside of you five days later. You will have to freeze your embryos and put them back inside of you a month later, when your ovaries have had time to calm down. I was given a paper with instructions of what to do, what to eat, when to start the ass shots, and what symptoms to look out for.

Due to the power outage at daycare, we were receiving email updates all day long about child care for the next day. The daycare center had planned to send Zoe to a sister center in Armonk, a town about fifteen minutes north of here, easy. The emails specifically said, "Check your email in the morning."

The next morning I woke up. I felt like shit. I felt as if I had been hit by a car, and then the driver of the car got out and kicked me repeatedly, in the lower stomach, while I was lying on the ground. It was horrible. I was beyond bloated. I looked pregnant – ironic. I could barely walk.

Should I take the day off? I can't with all of these fertility treatments for the past five months. I've taken too many days. A day for each IUI. A day for the HSG. Half a day for the IVF orientation class. I can't. I'll go in.

Without checking my email, I pack up Zoe and drive up to Armonk. I can barely lift her to get her in and out of her car seat. She is screaming and crying because she wants to be carried, and this time, I really cannot carry her. If I do pick her up, I risk upsetting my overly large ovaries. I can barely walk. Every step is sending shooting pains to all different parts of my body. I take small steps, and walk slowly, in an effort to not vibrate the rest of my body, because every step kills. We walk into the Armonk daycare, which looks like a beautiful ski chalet.

Damn.

"Hi, this is Zoe Jeffries. We're from the White Plains daycare center," I say nicely to the lady at the desk, cringing through my pain.

"Oh, good morning, they have their power back on, so you can drop her off there. I'm sorry," says the nicest person.

"FUUUUUUUUUCK!!!!" I scream so loud that it echoes off the ski chalet walls. "Sorry, it's okay, not your fault," and I turn around, and slowly walk out.

I put Zoe back into her car seat, tears welling up in my eyes from the pain. I speed off because now I am pissed off at myself, and I'm getting late. We drive to the White Plains daycare. We walk in, and I tell the director behind the desk that I went to Armonk by mistake. She feels badly for me, but she reminds me that I should have checked my email.

"Yeah, I know. I'm a freaking idiot, and have no one to blame but myself," I say, which is all true.

I drop Zoe off and head to work. I walk straight into my assistant principal's office. I slowly, with control, ease my body down to sit down in one of her chairs.

"So, I had my IVF retrieval yesterday," I say, "they took out thirty-three eggs."

"Wow," she says, "that's prolific." I think I understand what "prolific" means because of its context, but I make a mental note to look it up later, to make sure she is not insulting me.

"I really don't feel well. I can barely walk. I don't know if I will be able to make it through today," I confess to her, when what I really want to say is, *"I'm going to go home right now, because I can't move or walk."*

She explains to me that the entire third grade staff is out for math professional development, and that she would really appreciate it if I could hang in there because there are not enough substitutes to go around.

"Okay. I'll try," I say, which of course means, "I'll stay all day."

I start to walk down the long hallway to the stairwell, which leads to my room. I take the slowest and smallest steps I think I have ever taken in my life. It is noticeable. A second grade teacher comes out of her classroom and watches me – walking.

"You really look like you're not in a rush to get to your room," she says in her high-pitched second grade teacher voice.

Cut to Office Space: "Does someone have a case of the Mondays?"

"Ha!" I pretend laugh because her comment is not funny, "yeah, I guess so."

She continues to watch me walk as if I am either dying, or close to it. I pretend that this whole situation is normal. I get to my room and almost start to cry. I don't know if I can do this. I don't know if I can make it through today. I take a deep breath, and look up at the ceiling, so the tears do not start to fall down my face. Then, I start my regular pre-teaching morning routine.

I can do this. Fuck you IVF, I can do this.

I sit down at my computer, check my school email, and look up what the word "prolific" means.

After school, I rush home to rest for a whopping forty-five minutes before heading out to get Zoe from daycare.

Forty-five minutes, whoop-de-freakity-do.

I pick Zoe up at daycare. She still does not understand the concept that I cannot carry her. She is screaming, crying, and throwing herself on the floor.

Fuck me.

We get home and play a little. She eats dinner. I call the fertility clinic because I am in an exorbitant amount of pain and discomfort. Something has to be wrong. I leave a message with the service. We head upstairs for bath and nighttime routine. The doctor calls me back. I can tell by the voice that it is one of the female doctors who was often on call for the morning wanding sessions. There is something reassuring knowing that the woman on the other end of the phone has stuck a wand so far up my cooter that she could have spun me around the room.

I explain my symptoms to her, my pain, my discomfort. I question if I am experiencing that overhyperstimulation thing they warned me about.

Will this mean that I won't be able to put the embryos back inside of me on Saturday? Will I have to wait another whole month?

"What you're experiencing is very normal," she says. "It sucks, but it's totally normal. Your ovaries are extremely swollen and sensitive right now. You have to think about it like this: you had thirty-three eggs. That means the doctor stuck a needle into your ovaries thirty-three times to get each egg out. That's a lot, and your ovaries are reacting accordingly."

"Okay, it's Tuesday, what if these symptoms don't go away, then what?" I ask.

Planning, always planning.

"They most likely will, but if the symptoms don't go away, then we will have to consider freezing your embryos and putting them back inside of you next month," she explains.

We hang up. I do not want to wait another month. This process sucks. I just want it to be over. Zoe is losing her mind while I am on this quick phone call. I dry her off after the bath. She has a temper tantrum because I cannot carry her from the bathroom to her changing table, like normal. She needs to walk. She throws herself onto the floor. Brady is howling. Zoe is screaming. I am crying. Out of nowhere, my husband walks up the stairs.

Holy shit! He's home! He came home early. How did he know? Huge bonus points for him. Maybe even a blowjob when I feel better. Maybe. Probably not.

He takes over with Zoe and gets her to bed. I go to bed and cry. Going to work the day after the IVF retrieval was a mistake.

CHAPTER 12

Fresh Transfer – Putting the Egg Back In

We follow the directions and start the ass shots the following morning. They SUCK. It feels as though my husband took a sledgehammer and slammed it into my ass cheek. Then the following day, it feels the same on the other ass cheek. Then back to the first ass cheek.

Maybe I will look into starting those suppositories. How messy could it be?

I also start Estrogen patches. They are supposed to go on my stomach, but I am placing them more on my ass because I am going to Puerto Rico in a week, and no one wants to see my Estrogen patches peeking out from under my bathing suit.

The patches are what I would assume Nicotine patches are like. I do not feel them. I change them every other day. They are super sticky, and they are leaving a black line of sticky residue on my skin, and on my underwear. It is impossible to get the sticky stuff off. I would need to take a Brillo pad to my ass to get the sticky stuff off.

No thanks.

My symptoms after the IVF retrieval had subsided, which meant I was ready to get my embryo put back inside of me. It was Saturday, December 20th. John and I were, once again, at the fertility clinic. My mother-in-law was at my house watching Zoe.

The transfer was very similar to the retrieval in that I got into my scrubs and put my valuables into the locker. This time, there was less stress, no power outages, and normal blood pressure. John and I were sitting in that same little room where the woman had taken my vitals five days earlier and I had started sobbing uncontrollably. We sat down on the chairs, waiting to be told about the status of our embryos.

On Monday, they had taken out thirty-three eggs. Then, they put each individual egg into a petri dish with one sperm. The egg and the sperm meet each other in the dish and fertilize.

Swipe right egg and sperm. Swipe right.

There is also another procedure called ICSI, where the doctors actually put the sperm into the egg, but that is just for slower moving, stubborn sperm who cannot be bothered to ask for directions from the other side of the petri dish.

Over the past five days, my thirty-three eggs turned into into twenty-six fertilized embryos, and then by day five had turned into seventeen embryos. Seventeen day five blastocysts to be exact. The blastocyst is the embryo right at the point that it starts opening up from its cellular casing a little bit, which means it will stick better to my uterine lining, and maybe get me pregnant.

All I can think of are those little sponge capsule things we played with when we were little. They looked like a large antibiotic pill capsule, and when you put them in water, they start growing out of their capsule and turn into little sponge dinosaurs. I had seventeen little sponge dinosaurs.

The doctor explains to us how they grade the embryos by strength and viability. At this clinic, they do not give any "A's," but I had a number of very strong "B" grade embryos.

This seems totally fitting to me since "B" was typically the highest grade I ever got in school. Why would my embryos score any higher?

Then the doctor asked the question: "How many do you want to put back inside?"

My husband and I had talked about it on the drive down to the city that morning. "We should mess with the doctors and tell them that we want to put all seventeen back inside, and see what they say," John joked.

We decide to put one embryo back in.

I walk to the same surgery room where I walked into five days earlier. I hop up onto the table, legs in the air.

Say hello vagina!

The embryologist is right on the other side of the door. The doctors explain the embryos to me. They go through the whole, "this is your embryo, it is number and color coded unique to you," to make sure that I know that they are not putting someone else's baby inside of me.

The doctor gets prepared. She uses a sonogram, the type that they put on your stomach with the jelly, to see my uterus. She explains that she cannot use the wand because she is already in my vagina, with a tube inserting the embryo, and that would be a vaginal traffic jam. Literally.

New Yorkers understand traffic jams – regardless of the "jam" being with cars or vaginal canals – I get it.

I offer to hold the belly sonogram wand for her, because her hands seem full with the speculum, and the catheter, and inserting my future child. I like that I am holding it, it makes me feel in control, and as though I am part of the "baby making" equation, even though I am not at all.

When the doctor is ready, she yells out to the embryologist, who brings in my embryo and gives it to the doctor. The doctor sucks it out of the dish and shoots it up inside of me. I can see on the sonogram screen that she is placing it on the side of my uterus. She explains to me that if she places it there, then there is a more likely chance it will stick. The embryologist goes back to her room. We all stay still. The embryologist checks to make sure that the embryo is no longer in the dish.

"All clear!" Shouts the embryologist.

As I am standing up from the table, the embryologist walks over to me. "Here," she says, "for the baby book."

I look down. It is a picture of the embryo they just put inside of me.

"When did you take this?" I ask.

"Just right now, just before we put it inside of you," she says.

"Thank you," I say. I do not really know how to react. This is pretty cool, but I do not want to get my hopes up.

What if this doesn't work? What if there isn't a baby book?

I fold it up, put it inside of my purse, and do not look at it again until much later.

We get home. My sister-in-law and her boyfriend at the time are also visiting. I say a very brief hello and go upstairs to lie down. I feel totally fine. The transfer process is much like an IUI, painless, but I am exhausted. I am mentally, physically, emotionally, and vaginally exhausted. I sleep for hours. I wake up for dinner, and to be somewhat social to the family that is visiting. Although I do not know how socially acceptable I was that night given that most of the conversation revolved around how my doctor told me that my brain works exceptionally well on drugs. I am still boasting. Then I go back to sleep for the night.

Around two o'clock in the morning Zoe wakes up screaming. I run into her room. She is throwing up again, and again. She is so little that she does not even understand what throwing up means. She just does not "get" it, and she is very scared. John, my mother-in-law, and sister-in-law, all come in to help clean up the mess, while I am sitting in the chair trying to explain to my toddler that she needs to throw up into the Tupperware, not just straight into the towel. This concept is not going well. I scrap the Tupperware and just let her vomit again, and again, into the towel. I hold her tightly, and when it seems like she is done, I put her back to bed. The next day she is a wet noodle, sick as a dog, but not throwing up any longer.

That night, by ten o'clock, John starts vomiting like nothing I have ever heard before in my life. When he vomits, it sounds like his entire body becomes airborne, and then he lands, *slam*, on the ground. All I hear is vomit, *slam*, vomit, *and slam* for hours. I leave him to his vomiting and go downstairs to sleep far away from him.

Around three o'clock in the morning, I start having diarrhea. Insane jet propelling my ass off the toilet diarrhea. All of us are sick for the next few days. We were supposed to go to my parents' house for Christmas Eve dinner, but we skip it because we do not want to get my parents sick. On the phone with my mother, I tell her about the diarrhea.

"Mom, I think I shitted out my embryo," I tell her, dead seriously.

"You didn't shit out your embryo," she says.

"No, I really think I did. You have no idea how sick we all were. There is no way that embryo is still inside of me," I say emphatically.

"You do realize that is a totally different hole, correct?" She asks, because now she really thinks that I do not know the difference between the holes.

"Yeah Mah, I know it's a different hole," I say, "but still, this was a bad stomach bug, I would be shocked if my embryo is still in there."

In the meantime, I have started the progesterone suppositories that I requested in order to not have to do the ass shots. The suppositories are similar to a tampon applicator, but instead of shooting a tampon up inside of you, they shoot a cream pellet thing up inside of you. I was warned that it would be messy, and that I should wear a panty liner.

No fucking kidding. No one told me that maybe I should purchase stock in a panty liner company because I would use so many of them. Costco run?

The cream comes out of you naturally because of gravity right? No, we are not talking a little bit of cream here or there. We are talking chunks, upon chunks, upon chunks of cream falling out of me every minute. When I walk, move quickly, go to the bathroom. There are chunks of cream EVERYWHERE.

(What was that? I just lost the last male reader? Yup, that sounds about right.)

I would go to the bathroom, and the panty liner would be full of cream. I would wipe myself, and the toilet paper would be **full** of cream. I would stand up and flush, and the bowl would be **full** of cream. It was disgusting.

I asked for this? I requested this method of progesterone over the ass shots? Talk about a crappy six in one, and a shitty half dozen in the other. Both of these options suck donkey butt!

I made my husband wear condoms when we did have sex because I did not want any of this cream to get on his penis, and maybe into his bloodstream. One of us on IVF hormones was more than we could handle.

Would he start growing boobs? Who knows?

Christmas morning, Thursday, December 25, 2014, I wake up early because we are catching a plane to Puerto Rico. My boobs hurt like hell.

Holy Shit! I'm pregnant! I think to myself. *No, don't get excited. This could be the infertility mind fuck. These could be false symptoms. But it's not. I know it's not. I never had sore boobs before. I really think I'm pregnant.*

We meet my sister, and her family, in Puerto Rico. I briefly explain IVF to my teenage step-niece and nephew, and forewarn them that in three days I am supposed to take a pregnancy test. At which point, I will either drink my face off (exact words) if it is negative, or I will be pregnant.

Our vacation is going great. I have not slept a wink since we got to Puerto Rico because I am obsessing about the fact that I might be pregnant. Obsessing. Monday morning rolls around, and I take a pregnancy test in the hotel bathroom. I have to wait for John to finish having diarrhea because he is still reaping the benefits of the stomach virus from a week ago.

It's POSITIVE!!! I'm pregnant!

Apparently, I didn't shit out my embryo – good to know.

I am supposed to go to any blood lab clinic to confirm that I am in fact pregnant, and to check my progesterone and estrogen levels. I try to go to a Quest Lab in Puerto Rico, but after taking a taxi there and back, I find out that I need a certain type of order from the doctor back home.

Finally, after many missed calls, I tell the fertility clinic back in New York that I will go into their clinic the morning that I am back home. The way I see it, if I am still pregnant at that point, then I will still be pregnant, and if my levels are bad and something happens before then, that it is totally out of my control.

We have an excellent vacation, minus the suppository cream falling out of me and chunking into my bathing suit and underwear. Every move I make cream is chunking, and chunking. Chunking.

CHAPTER 13

I Laid a Dinosaur Egg

We return to New York, and confirm the pregnancy at the clinic. I am still on the estrogen patches, and the suppositories, chunk, chunk. I am still going into the clinic, but now it is once a week, to check my levels. They are making sure the HCG is going up, and the progesterone and estrogen are at the right levels. After week eight of the pregnancy, I am transferred to my regular ob-gyn, but still being monitored by the clinic. It is not until week twelve that the clinic starts my "step down" protocol, which is code for the way they want me to wean my body off the progesterone suppositories and the estrogen patches. Little by little, I stop using the suppositories and the patches, and now I am just pregnant, a normal pregnancy. The cream did not stop chunking out of me until week fifteen, which I found impressive.

Way to hang in there as long as you can cream, I thought to myself.

This pregnancy continues normally, aside from the fact that I gain weight so rapidly that I am shocked at every doctor appointment. I carry my second daughter until 41 weeks of pregnancy. Again, I cannot get pregnant, but once I am pregnant, I carry my daughters for as long as a person is medically permitted to be pregnant.

I am forty weeks pregnant. My due date has come and gone. I am at the doctor's office for my weekly check-up. He is doing the ultrasound; I can see my baby on the screen. I can feel her inside of me. For the past few weeks, I have been watching the black pockets of amniotic fluid get smaller and smaller on the screen, this time they look very small.

"Alright, come back in a week," says the doctor who I do not like anymore.

"Come back in a week?" I question, "What about the amniotic fluid?"

"Yeah, it seems fine, come back in a week."

Alrighty.

I am suspicious, but I do as the doctor tells me. I return to the ob-gyn a week later. Still pregnant. My regular doctor is out of the office for Rosh Hashanah. I think he is Jewish, but I might have made that up. I am sitting on the ob-gyn table, drape covering my vagina, waiting for this other doctor who I have never met before to come in. John is with me. He is working from home this week since I am supposed to be having a baby any day now, although I do not think the baby was copied on that email memo.

The new doctor walks in and says, "Alright, let's see what's going on with the va-jay-jay." I **immediately** like her.

**Cut to My Cousin Vinny - In the courtroom, when the other lawyer is stuttering and Vinny knocks it out of the park, and the defendant friend stands up and screams: "I want him!" **

I make a mental note to switch to this female doctor as soon as I can. This woman speaks my language.

She does an internal exam. "All good," she says.

"You're not going to do an ultrasound?" I ask.

"When was your last ultrasound?" she asks me.

"A week ago," I explain to her, almost at the point of demanding.

"A week ago?!" she exclaims. "Yes you're right we need to do one now, that's abnormal. Normally when a patient is overdue, we do two ultrasounds a week."

I look over at my husband, the lawyer, who is making a mental note that if anything is wrong with this baby, he is going to sue everyone he can. She gets out the jelly, and starts moving the camera over my ginormous belly. As she is moving the ultrasound all around I say, "See, I am seeing pockets of fluid, but I'm not seeing a pocket that doesn't have umbilical cord also in it," (which I know from talking to my other doctor does not count as an amniotic fluid pocket).

"Are you an ultrasound technician?" she asks me.

"No, I teach fourth grade," I say.

"So you just Google a lot?" she asks.

"No," I say, "I can just see it. It just makes sense to me."

"Well, alright, you have no fluid left. You're going to the hospital and having this baby today," she says.

We leave, go home, get Zoe from daycare, have my parents come and watch her until my mother-in-law arrives from Boston, and we head to the hospital. I am admitted.

John and I are in the delivery room, and in walks this very normal looking guy wearing normal clothes.

"Hey, I'm Josh. Josh Whiteman," (not his real last name) he shakes my hand hard.

"Hi?" I say in a questioning tone, because I have no idea who this guy is.

He moves my purse and takes a seat in one of the supplied hospital chairs. "So, do you know why you're here?" He asks me, sitting there with his legs crossed, as if we are having beers. I still do not know who this guy is, or what his role is.

"To have a baby? I think?" I say.

"Right. Yes, that. You also have no fluid left inside of you, so we're going to get you started on Cervidil. Did the nurses explain this to you?"

"Yes."

Who is this man?

"They told me that Cervidil is a patch, which is inserted into the cervix to start contractions, kind of like Pitocin."

"That's right!" he says excitedly.

No, seriously people. Who the ***fuck*** *is this guy?*

He explains that he is going to do an internal, just to check how far along my cervix feels.

Fine, totally fine. I think to myself. *I've have many internals, no big deal.*

I was wrong. He gloves up, and sticks his entire arm up inside of me. He is elbow deep in my vagina. I quickly grab the railings of the hospital bed because he is so far up inside of me, that I think my head is going to hit the wall behind me. I immediately think that he must have put the wrong gloves on. He needs those veterinarian gloves that go all the way up to your elbow. The type Billy Crystal did not have in *City Slickers* when he lost his watch pulling Norman, the cow, out of Norman's mother.

This guy is totally going to lose his watch inside of me.

I look over at John. His jaw is dropped and his eyes are wide open. He is smiling, but only because he thinks this whole situation is completely unbelievable. Dr. Whiteman retracts his arm, which takes forever. In my head, I am hearing the beeping sounds of a Mac truck backing up. He then asks me how much I think the baby weighs.

"I don't know," I say, "no one mentioned that to me."

Without skipping a beat, Dr. Whiteman grabs my belly from the outside, and starts roughly, and aggressively, moving it around, as though he was holding a basketball, and bouncing it from one hand to the other. I, again, grab hold of the railings.

I'm going to fall out of this bed. I think to myself. *Holy crap! This is painful. Is he this rough when he's having sex?*

"Ehhh," he says, while jostling my belly and me, "I think it's a good seven pound baby, not too big. You'll be good."

I'll be good? I don't know if I'll ever be the same after that exam. Who **is** *this guy?*

"Alright," he continues, "I'm going to let the nurses get to it, you're in good hands."

He leaves.

John looks at me, "Who was that guy?" he asks.

"I don't really know. I think he's our doctor?" I say, totally confused. For all I knew, he was a very handsy financial advisor.

John Googles his name and, yes, it turns out he is our doctor. Our doctor cross covers with another medical practice, and we had never seen this guy before.

Phew, that's a relief. Otherwise that would have been such a bizarre encounter.

They insert the Cervidil patch into my vagina. A few hours later, the contractions get strong. I get my epidural. Around twelve-thirty in the morning a bunch of nurses start to come into my room. I feel a lot of pressure, as if I need to take a large crap.

They ask me to do a practice push to see if I am a good "pusher." I am feeling judged. I do a practice push. Apparently, I am an all right pusher. Now, I am starting to actually push. After my first real push, the nurse starts screaming, "It's in the sac!!! It's in the sac!!" and she looks at the doctor for advice on what to do next.

What?!?!?

"What does that mean?" I ask, totally panicking. "Is that okay?"

He looks up at me from inside my vagina, "It's totally fine," he says calmly. "It's perfectly healthy. It's just very rare, and very cool."

I had no amniotic fluid left, so my water never broke, so the "bag" never broke.

Very cool? I think to myself. *What?*

I do one more push and out comes what looks to me like a baby in a condom. My baby was on the table, completely encased in a clear condom-looking bag.

Am I a dinosaur? Did I just lay an egg?

The doctor then took his fingers, popped open the bag, and out came my daughter.

WHAT THE FUCK WAS THAT?!?!

They put my newly born "sac baby" on my chest. This moment was such a magical and rare birth event, the nurses were all talking about it.

Once I had determined that enough time had passed after this amazing, one in eighty-thousand, "sac baby" birth experience – forty-five seconds later – I turn to the nurse and ask, "Did I poop?"

She shakes her head at me, in a combination of disdain and disapproval, and says, "No, sweetie. You didn't poop."

The End

AFTERWORD

Hi! I am Karen, and I am infertile! I am the creator of the Hilariously Infertile platform, including the website, book and social media accounts. How did this all come to be? Sometimes I ask myself that exact same question.

I was on maternity leave with my "sac baby" and I was helping a few friends through their infertility "journeys." I was telling my husband one night, "Well, Jessica said her follicles were at 17 milimeters, so she will have her IUI on Sunday, and Allison said that she is ovulating right now, so it is 'go' time for them."

Aside from the fact that my husband did not see it necessary to know all of my friends' ovulation schedules, he said, "You should write a book."

I joked at how ridiculous that sounded. He retorted, "I am being serious. A self-help book for women who are going through this. You are helping your friends. Maybe you could help other people too?"

I laughed it off and thought nothing of it. A few weeks later during a naptime, I just opened up my laptop and started writing. I had no idea what I was writing, I was just writing about all of it. It was cathartic and helpful, and all of the sudden I realized, *Holy shit, this is funny!*

I knew that my take on infertility was humorous. I showed it to my friend, Gillian, first. I asked her what she thought about it. I asked her what she thought it *was*. Was it a book? Was it a blog? Was it just me journaling about my "journey?"

She told me she had no idea what it *was*, but that I should not stop. "Keep going," she said, "who knows what it is, and it doesn't matter, just keep going." I am so thankful for those words.

I kept writing. The more I wrote, the more I laughed at what I wrote, and the more I gained confidence and strength to show it to other people. I showed it to my husband next.

"Not exactly the self-help book I had in mind," he said in an almost scolding, and totally judging tone, "but I really like it, and yes, keep going."

So I kept writing. About six weeks later I had, what is now, *Hilariously Infertile* the book. What do I do now?

In my naiveté, I just thought that once you write a book, you send it to some publishers, and then they publish your work. I didn't realized that you usually have to be famous to get your book published.

I was emailing people all day long, sending them my horribly drafted query letter. I heard very little in response. The replies that I did receive all said the same thing, "We just don't think this is a big enough market."

That enraged me! Not a big enough market? Not a big enough market? It is, in fact, one of the fastest growing medical fields in the United States. The statistics are staggering. Then I realized, no one thinks it is a big enough market, because no one is talking about it, and definitely, no one is laughing about it. It was then that I made it my mission to prove to the world that we can, and we should, be talking openly, frankly, honestly, and humorously about infertility, because no one deserves to be suffering quietly in the dark.

I was still super bummed about not getting a publisher in the first two months of trying, haha, but I got over it. A friend suggested that I start my own website and social media platform. I was skeptical. I am a school teacher. I never had a personal Facebook account and now I was going to have a website?

I looked into it. I started designing the website and created the social media accounts. My niece, Natalie, explained what a hashtag is to me, and the rest is history – or, at least, completely documented on my social media.

At every turn since Hilariously Infertile's inception I have said, "If this is how far it gets, I am happy with that."

If responding to this one person is all that I did for the world – that is good. If responding to hundreds of people is all I did for the world – that is good. If keeping in touch with hundreds of my thousands of followers is all I do for the world – that is good. I was ready, at each step, to understand that each step might be the last step, and yet, it kept going.

Now, about you guys. The stories that I have been humbled to hear from my followers are the most incredibly amazing stories I have heard in my life – stories about loss, tragedy, love, persistence, power, heartbreak, detriment and above all else, the strength of the human will. I am beyond humbled by this experience, and I hope that I can continue to make everyone laugh a little bit during such a sorrowful time in your lives.

We will cry. We will scream. We will fall down, and we will get up and move forward in whatever direction we choose, given what life has put in front of us. However, and I hate to sound too much like *Footloose* here but, we will **fucking laugh** about it when we can!

SPECIAL THANKS:

There are so many people to thank. First, I would like to thank my husband, who's real name is **Jeffrey**, for being beyond supportive of me while I share everything about my vagina with the world. It was Jeff's idea to start writing the book, and he supported me every step of the way. Also, to **my beautiful daughters** who make me smile every day. I hope that you never have to go through infertility if you want to have children, but if you do, you came to the right place.

To **my parents** and mostly my sister, **Katie**, who at first were confused by what I was doing, thank you for supporting me through my own infertility and also through the conception and development of Hilariously Infertile. Katie, you are not only my sister you are my best friend, I have looked up to you since I can remember (until I got taller and started looking down to you). You have always supported me and listened to me no matter what, and I am so thankful for that.

To **my in-laws**, there are **so** many of you, thank you for always accepting me for who and what I am, you are the best family that a girl could marry into.

To **Robyn**, my best friend since college, thank you for always taking the time to listen to me regardless of what is going on in your life, we are life-long friends and I love that. You are wise beyond your years, Robyn, and I am so lucky to have you in my life.

To **Allison** and **Justin**, I really don't know how to thank you both enough for all of your love and support. Allison, you supported me through my infertility and I hope I did the same for you. I never had to worry about what to say or think around you, because you are the best, selfless, non judging friend, that anyone could have. Justin, you believed in Hilariously Infertile: the platform, before it even was a platform, you saw the potential and pushed me to get out there and post more. You believed that this could be huge before it was anything, you not only knew that the message was important, but you believed that I was the right person to send that message to people, thank you for that.

To **Gillian**, thank goodness I sent you that first copy of the book over two years ago, and thank goodness you told me to keep writing. I didn't know what I was doing, but I knew that you, a good friend, an avid reader, and one of the smartest most worldly people I know, liked it and told me to keep going. That was all I needed, and that was everything.

Natalie, you have been a part of *Hilariously Infertile* since the first month, without you, I wouldn't know what a hashtag is. You are brilliant and creative, and such an asset to whatever company you land at. It has been a joy to watch you and your brother grow up for the past decade, it is my hope that my children will turn out to be a mere fraction of the amazing people you and Dylan are. If my children can even achieve that, I will be happy, because you and Dylan are incredible. Thank you for all your hard work, this book, the social media, the whole platform would have failed if not for you.